BWB Texts

Short books on big subjects from great New Zealand writers

Antibiotic Resistance
The End of Modern Medicine?

SIOUXSIE WILES

Published in 2017 by Bridget Williams Books Limited, PO Box 12474, Wellington 6144, New Zealand, www.bwb.co.nz, info@bwb.co.nz.

© Siouxsie Wiles 2017

This BWB Text is copyright. Apart from fair dealing for the purpose of private study, research, criticism or review, permitted under the Copyright Act, no part may be reproduced by any process without the prior permission of the copyright holder and the publisher.

ISBN 9780947518653 (Paperback), ISBN 9780947518660 (EPUB)
ISBN 9780947518677 (Kindle), ISBN 9780947518684 (PDF)
DOI 10.7810/9780947518653

A catalogue record for this book is available from the National Library of New Zealand. Kei te pātenga raraunga o Te Puna Mātauranga o Aotearoa te whakarārangi o tēnei pukapuka

Acknowledgements
The publisher acknowledges the ongoing support provided by the Bridget Williams Books Publishing Trust and Creative New Zealand.

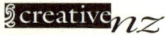

Publisher: Tom Rennie
Editors: Geoff Walker and Denis Welch
Cover and internal design: Base Two
Typesetter: Tina Delceg
Printer: Printlink, Wellington

CONTENTS

Introduction	7
1. A miscellany of microbes	9
2. Infectious diseases around the world and in New Zealand	21
3. A new era of medicine dawns	37
4. Antimicrobial resistance	46
5. How antibiotics are used	54
6. Antibiotic use in New Zealand	66
7. The threats to New Zealand from antibiotic resistance	76
8. Time for action	93
List of acronyms	111
Appendix: Quiz answers from page 15	113
Notes	117
About the author	130
Acknowledgements	131
About BWB Texts	133

INTRODUCTION

Bacteria, viruses, fungi, parasites. Do you know the difference? These microorganisms live, mostly hidden and unseen, on our skin, up our noses, and in our guts. They're also on our pets and livestock, and among plants, rivers and soils – in virtually every place on Earth you can think of. The vast majority of them are completely harmless. Some are even beneficial, degrading dead matter, recycling nutrients, and producing delicious cheeses and intoxicating beverages.

A small number, though, can cause devastation to human and animal health, our environment, and our economy. It's these that I became fascinated with when, as a teenager, I first picked up a book called *The Fireside Book of Deadly Diseases* by Robert Wilkins. Little did I know that Wilkins's book would set me on my path to become a microbiologist, on a mission to understand how infectious microbes make us sick and how we can stop them.

Like so much in life, it's complicated. There is no single threat or one-size-fits-all solution. But the experts do all agree on one thing: we are running out of ways to treat infectious microorganisms and the diseases they cause. The prediction is that, without urgent action, by 2025 we could see a return to the pre-antibiotic era when a simple stubbed toe could mean amputation or death.

Untreatable strains of infectious microbes are already circulating around the world and causing incurable disease. But it's not just our ability to treat infectious diseases that's at risk. It's modern medicine as a whole. Many life-saving and routine medical procedures and treatments rely on us being able to prevent infection: organ transplants, chemotherapy for cancer, knee and hip replacements, to name just a few. In a world without effective antibiotics, even routine surgery will become life-threateningly risky once again.

In this book, I'll introduce you to the world of infectious microorganisms, explain the growing burden they place on us here in Aotearoa New Zealand, and outline the very real threats we face from antibiotic resistance. Brace yourself.

1. A MISCELLANY OF MICROBES

Many scientists, myself included, get very upset when TV or radio newsreaders and newspaper articles describe bacteria as viruses or vice versa. It probably looks like we're being pedantic. To most people, viruses and bacteria are, if not the same, at least very similar. But they are not. Understanding how different microorganisms survive in the first place is fundamental to our ability to treat the diseases they cause. Let me introduce you to the diverse world of microbes.

BACTERIA: HERE, THERE AND EVERYWHERE

Bacteria are microscopic, ranging in size from 0.5 to 5 microns. For comparison, human cells range from 7 to 120 microns in diameter. One micron is one-millionth of a metre. If you took a cube the size of a grain of salt, you would be able to fit more than 15 million bacteria into it. That's more than three times the number of people who live in New Zealand. Bacteria are made up of a gooey substance called cytoplasm. This is where all their biochemical processes take place, regulated by the particular set of genetic instructions encoded by their DNA (deoxyribonucleic acid).

To keep their cytoplasm from oozing all over the place, bacteria are surrounded by a cell membrane and a mesh-like layer of sugars and amino acids called peptidoglycan. Some also have a second membrane layer around their peptidoglycan.[1] A few cover themselves with fatty acids instead, while others produce a viscous layer of slime. These differences make some bacteria harder to kill than others. In some cases, much, much harder. I'll come back to that later.

Bacteria reproduce by splitting in two, but the time taken to do this can vary widely. Some split every 20–30 minutes, turning one bacterium into several million in 10 hours. Others reproduce at a more leisurely pace, taking days or weeks to divide. If the conditions for growth aren't quite right, some bacteria turn into spores, which are almost indestructible little versions of themselves. Spores can survive dormant for years.

In short, bacteria are alive, have their own metabolism, feed from their environment, and reproduce. Some even have a sort of motorised tail, called a flagellum, that they use like an outboard motor, enabling them to swim. Bacteria live in almost every environment on Earth, from Antarctic soils and the hot springs of Rotorua, to your bellybutton and nose. Estimates vary, but it's thought that there are at least as many, if not more, bacterial cells living in and on us, as there are living cells of our own body.[2]

VIRUSES: CUCKOOS IN THE NEST

Compared to bacteria, viruses are much simpler and much, much smaller, measuring between 0.02 and 0.2 microns. If you took your grain-of-salt-sized cube, you would be able to fit 125 billion viruses into it. That's more than 17 times the world's human population.

Viruses are made up of an outer shell (called a capsid) surrounding their genetic material, which can be either DNA or RNA (ribonucleic acid). They don't have any gooey cytoplasm, so can't carry out any biochemical reactions. Instead, they rely on the energy, chemicals and machinery of their 'host' – a susceptible cell of a higher organism.

Strictly speaking, viruses aren't alive. Once one is taken up by its host cell, it hijacks the cell and gets it to read the virus's genetic material; the cell will then start replicating the virus. This can end in disaster for the host cell, which is often destroyed when burst open by the new viruses.

Some viruses are less brutal, budding off their host cell's membrane but leaving the cell intact. Some 'genetically engineer' their hosts instead, incorporating their genetic material into the host's genome in the ultimate form of immortality.

In summary, viruses are just packaged code waiting for a host cell to translate and replicate. Unlike bacteria, they don't have their own metabolism. Instead, they rely on invading other organisms to survive and reproduce. Depending on the virus, hosts can be humans, animals, plants and even bacteria. Again, estimates vary, but it's thought that a teaspoon of seawater contains as many as five million viruses.

FUNGI: THE WORLD'S GREAT DECOMPOSERS

Next up, fungi. Who isn't familiar with yeasts, moulds and mushrooms? These are all types of fungi, which belong to a kingdom of life all their own, distinct from plants, animals and bacteria. Fungal cells range in size from 5 to 30 microns in diameter. Their cell walls contain chitin, a very strong derivative of sugar also found in the exoskeletons of insects and crustaceans.

Yeasts live as single cells and can reproduce by either splitting in two or by mating with another yeast. They can convert carbohydrates to alcohol and carbon dioxide through fermentation, something we've been exploiting for thousands of years to make bread, wine and beer.

Moulds grow as multicellular filaments called hyphae, which are like the fungal version of a plant's roots or branches. The hyphae emit enzymes to break down nearby food, which could be the cellulose in your bathroom wall or the lignin in tree bark, and then absorb the resulting nutrients. Fungi can grow a massive network of hyphae known as a mycelium.[3]

Mushrooms are the fruiting bodies of many fungi. Within their gills are millions of tiny reproductive cells, confusingly also called spores, that germinate to form hyphae when they find themselves in the right conditions. Many fungi have spores evolved to be dispersed by the wind, but others have more interesting ways of getting around, such as producing a stinky slime to attract flies.

In summary, fungi – like bacteria – are alive, have their own metabolism, feed from their environment, and reproduce. Found in every environment on Earth, they are nature's great recyclers. They decompose organic matter like plants and animals, releasing vital nutrients that are then used by plants and other organisms to grow.

PARASITES: VERY ATTACHED TO YOU

Finally, we have parasites, defined as organisms that live on or in a host organism and get their food from or at the expense of their host. Three main types can cause disease in humans: protozoa, helminths and ectoparasites.

Protozoa are single-celled organisms that behave like animals. They are mostly microscopic, up to 150 microns in size. If you took your grain-of-salt-sized cube one last time, you would be able to fit about 37 of those 150-micron-sized parasites into it.

Like bacteria, they are made up of cytoplasm surrounded by a cell membrane, although some are also covered in an outer surface called a pellicle. Unlike bacteria, but similar to humans and animals, protozoan cytoplasm contains 'organelles' in which critical biological processes are carried out, and their DNA is contained in a nucleus enclosed by a membrane. Some protozoa have a sort of mouth (called a cytosome) for ingesting fluids or solid particles, and many protozoa can move around, either by using their flagella tails or waving hair-like cilia, or by means that I can only describe as 'oozing'.

Helminths are unrelated large, multicellular worm-like organisms generally visible to the naked eye in the adult stage of their life cycle. Those capable of causing disease in humans include flukes, tapeworms, thorny-headed worms and roundworms. Flukes have a pair of distinctive-looking suckers, and tapeworms can grow more than 15 metres long. Thorny-headed worms have a proboscis armed with hooks that they use to attach themselves to their host's tissues. Roundworms are usually round with a shield-shaped head.

Helminths reproduce by laying as many as hundreds of thousands of eggs at a time, generally once a day but sometimes more often. These eggs hatch out into larvae that mature into adults that can live for years. Some helminths are hermaphrodites, while others have males and females.

Lastly, the term *ectoparasite* generally refers to organisms like ticks, fleas, lice and mites that attach to or burrow into their host's skin. They can cause diseases in their own right but are even more important as transmitters of other microorganisms.

So, do you know your bacterial diseases from your viral infections? Or how about fungi from parasites? Take a guess at what some of these diseases are caused by: tuberculosis (TB), AIDS, botulism, bilharzia, impetigo, pneumonia, measles, syphilis, gonorrhoea, toxoplasmosis, meningitis, polio, influenza, rheumatic fever, tonsillitis, aspergillosis, malaria, ringworm. Or how about these microorganisms: MRSA, Zika, HIV, *Campylobacter jejuni*, hepatitis A, *Giardia lamblia*, *Staphylococcus aureus*, *Chlamydia trachomatis*, *Haemophilus influenzae*.[4] The answers are at the back of the book.

PROTECTING OURSELVES

The World Health Organization (WHO) defines infectious diseases as diseases caused by microorganisms that can be spread, directly or indirectly, from one person to another. This includes zoonotic diseases transmitted from animals to humans. We encounter infectious microorganisms all the time, but we've evolved defences to deal with them. Our immune system is made up of lots of different cells and organs designed to recognise and neutralise threats.

We can divide these defences into two broad categories, one of which is non-specific but very fast (our innate immune system), and the other of which is slower but more specific (our adaptive immune system). A key feature of the latter is that it can 'remember' what it encounters so that it can react faster the next time it sees the same threat.

Vaccination is the best way of preventing infectious diseases. Here we get our body to generate 'memory' by exposing ourselves to either a deactivated version or a tiny part of a microorganism. This equips our immune system with the tools it needs to beat the microorganism when we next meet the real deal. The simpler a microorganism's structure, the easier it is to develop a vaccine, so this strategy has been most effective for viruses.

Honestly, if you are a healthy person with no underlying medical conditions, always get vaccinated. Not only will you protect yourself against the disease but you'll be contributing to 'herd immunity'. This protects those in your community who are unable to be vaccinated by reducing the number of susceptible people spreading the disease around.

The problem with vaccination is that, at the moment, it's not possible to make vaccines for all infectious diseases. In some cases, this is because we don't know which bits of the microorganisms we have to show our immune system so that it recognises the organism in future. For more wily microorganisms, it's because they mimic parts of our body to hide from us during infection. The last thing we want to do is create a vaccine that attacks our own body.

The fact that some microorganisms come in hundreds of different versions makes it difficult to produce a vaccine that can protect against all variants. The influenza virus, for instance, evolves so fast that each year the flu vaccine has to be reformulated.

Another way of protecting ourselves and other people from infectious diseases is by making small changes to our behaviour. Like washing our hands properly, using condoms, and not swimming in rivers and lakes that may contain infectious microorganisms. We can also take care not to consume raw milk, unwashed fruits and veggies, or undercooked meat. But it's hard to imagine us all wearing face masks (and I don't mean those flimsy little paper things you sometimes see people wearing) to stop breathing in the infectious microorganisms floating around in the air. Did you know that a single sneeze expels tens of thousands of saliva droplets, some of which remain airborne indefinitely? This is a big problem when they may also be teeming with infectious microorganisms.

TREATING INFECTIOUS DISEASES

The generic word for something that can stop the growth of, or kill, a microorganism is 'antimicrobial'. For bacteria, fungi and parasites, the main way we do this is by trying to disrupt their cell membranes and biochemical processes, which can either kill them outright or just stop them growing while our immune system deals with them. This strategy works quite well for bacteria. They are different enough from us that the more modern drugs we use either don't affect us much or at all. Antimicrobial agents that target bacteria are called antibacterials or antibiotics, and they only work against particular bacteria. Similarly, agents that target fungi are known as antifungals and they only work against particular fungi.

Parasites are targeted with drugs called antiparasitics, but because parasites are more like us than bacteria are, we have fewer options for treating them. And the drugs that target viruses (antivirals) don't work against all viruses, because the host–virus interaction is usually very specific. As these interactions don't exist when the host cell is going about its usual business, antivirals shouldn't affect normal host cells either.

Even with effective medicines, treatment is often complicated by the fact that the symptoms of many infections are indistinguishable. Telling them apart is a major problem that scientists are trying to solve, because correct diagnosis and rapid treatment can make the difference between life and death.

Got a rash? Well, that could be a mild viral infection or infection with meningococcal bacteria, which could kill you in a few hours if you aren't treated with the right antibiotics. Got a chesty cough? That could be a sign of bacterial pneumonia or viral bronchitis.

A friend of mine who's a paediatrician has described the anguish of seeing sick children and knowing it'll be days before they find out what is making them sick. Take the case of 'Toby', an eight-week-old boy who had become unwell very quickly. When my friend saw him he had a high fever, was dehydrated and looked very sick. My friend was in no doubt that Toby had an infection, but what was it? Would antibiotics help? Which would be best? Or was it a viral infection that would get better by itself if they just provided supportive care like food, fluid and pain relief?

My friend took some blood and did a lumbar puncture to sample the fluid that flows around Toby's brain and sent them to the lab to look for signs of blood infection or meningitis. But it takes several days to reliably tell if there is no infection, and children as young as Toby can deteriorate and die very quickly if they've got a bacterial infection. So my friend started treatment with a combination of antibiotics that would kill a wide range of different bacteria. Toby improved, no bacteria grew from his samples, and two days later he went home. A good outcome.

But right from the start my friend knew that Toby probably had a viral infection. Ninety-five per cent of 'Tobys' do. This means that for every twenty sick kids like that, only one really needs antibiotics. My friend made the right treatment decision, because until the tests come back, you just can't tell which baby's life is at risk from a bacterial infection. Indeed, this is the approach that our national guidelines recommend. But my friend, and all the other doctors like them, are also contributing to a worldwide crisis that threatens modern medicine. By the end of this book, you'll understand why it's so crucial that scientists develop better ways of preventing, diagnosing and treating infectious diseases.

2. INFECTIOUS DISEASES AROUND THE WORLD AND IN NEW ZEALAND

Now that you have met the many different types of infectious microbes, I want to explain how they impact on human health. The facts are at our fingertips, thanks to the Global Burden of Diseases Study funded by the Bill and Melinda Gates Foundation, where you'll find all the information on what people have died of since 1990. It's available on a website for anyone to explore.[1] If you are curious, you can pick a region or country and see how the causes of death there have changed over the past twenty years or so.

In 2015, infectious diseases caused 8.1 million deaths globally, a little over one in ten of the total deaths that year. Infectious microbes killed almost as many people that year as cancer (8.7 million). The leading cause was cardiovascular disease, with almost 18 million deaths worldwide.

Studies like this tend, however, to under-represent the number of people who die from infectious diseases. They only allow for one cause of death per person, and often this is recorded as the underlying disease a person had, rather than the immediate cause of death. For example, many of those recorded as having died of a neurological condition like Alzheimer's will probably have died of pneumonia or a urinary tract infection.

In countries with the lowest incomes, infectious diseases were the leading reason why people died in 2015, responsible for more than two-fifths of all deaths. But before you start thinking of infectious diseases as a 'Third World' problem, you might be surprised to learn that deaths from 'diarrhoea, lower respiratory tract infections, and other common infectious diseases' ranked sixth for high-income countries. But this still doesn't tell the whole story of the burden of infectious diseases. To do that, we need to dig deeper into a different dataset – the reasons why people are admitted to hospital.

WE'RE BUCKING INTERNATIONAL TRENDS, BUT NOT IN A GOOD WAY

The global study shows that as countries become more developed their rates of infectious diseases fall, and their rates of non-communicable diseases like cancer rise as people live longer. I was astonished when I found out that here in New Zealand we are heading in the other direction. Our rates for many infectious diseases are going up, not down. When Professor Michael Baker and his colleagues studied the reasons people were admitted to hospital,[2] they found that the number of overnight admissions due to non-communicable diseases had risen by 7 per cent in twenty years. No surprises there. The shocking finding was that the number of overnight admissions due to infectious diseases had gone up by a staggering 50 per cent!

In the year July 2013 to June 2014, almost 91 thousand Kiwis had infectious diseases listed as the primary reason for being hospitalised, accounting for around 8 per cent of all hospitalisations that year.[3] That number jumps to 25 per cent – one in four – when we look at admissions where patients end up staying at least overnight. And many other people in hospital will also be battling an infectious disease as a result of having a compromised immune system. This might be because they've had surgery, or they have a non-communicable disease like cancer or diabetes. These people won't feature in the numbers, though, as their underlying disease would be listed as the primary cause of hospitalisation.

Fortunately, most of the infectious diseases to which New Zealanders are exposed are still treatable. Just over 1,200 or about 4 per cent of the 29,636 people who died in 2013 had infectious diseases listed as the primary cause of their demise.[4] Unfortunately, for reasons I'll explain later, many of these diseases are becoming very difficult to treat.

In 2013, over two-thirds of our infectious disease hospitalisations were for bacterial infections.[5] The major culprits were *Staphylococcus aureus*, *Streptococcus pyogenes*, and food and water-borne infections caused by a variety of organisms.[6] Let's take a closer look at these foes.

FROM HARMLESS COMPANION TO FATAL ADVERSARY

Staphylococcus aureus is probably more commonly known as 'staph' and is one of the bacteria that comes in hundreds of different varieties, which is why we still don't have an effective vaccine to protect against it. This organism really is a 'superbug'. It's massive repertoire of genes enables it to cause a wide variety of illness, from nasty boils and food poisoning to pneumonia, meningitis, and blood poisoning (bacteraemia).

For the women reading this, *S. aureus* is one of the reasons you are told to regularly change tampons during your period. It can produce a toxin that switches your immune system into hyperdrive. The disease this can cause, toxic shock syndrome, is very rare, but fatal if not treated quickly. About a third of healthy people carry *S. aureus*, usually in their nose and throat, and sometimes on their skin or in their intestines. This is one of the main reasons for those alcohol gel dispensers you are supposed to use when visiting someone in hospital.

Picture the scene: an elderly relative has fallen and ended up in hospital. You're taking them some flowers and grapes to cheer them up. The flowers make your nose a little itchy so you give it a scratch. You're in a rush and forget to use the hand gel. You deposit a nice splodge of *S. aureus* on their glass when they ask you for a drink of water. They pick up the glass – and possibly a nasty infection.

S. aureus is very good at lurking around in our environment, too, on places like door handles, taps and computer keyboards. It's also incredibly adept at colonising medical devices like catheters and artificial joints. When a piece of plastic or metal is inserted in your body, it very quickly becomes covered in special molecules we make called proteins. *S. aureus* has a huge number of its own proteins that recognise and bind to our proteins, allowing them to tether themselves to the inserted device. The bacteria then grow into a little community called a biofilm, surrounded by a sticky goo that protects them from antibiotics and our immune system.

Time for some numbers. Dr Deborah Williamson is a medically qualified microbiologist who, along with Michael Baker, has spearheaded recent efforts to calculate the burden of several infectious diseases in New Zealand. The findings make grim reading. First, our rates of *S. aureus* disease are the highest in the developed world – and rising. Between 2000 and 2011, over 61 thousand people were hospitalised for an *S. aureus* infection.[7] The vast majority of these cases (about 85 per cent) were related to skin and soft tissue infections; 11 per cent were due to bacteraemia and 4 per cent to pneumonia. The people more likely to have skin and soft tissue infections were children under five, while cases of bacteraemia or pneumonia were more likely in people over seventy. A study focused on what happened to 134 hospital patients who had *S. aureus* bacteraemia between June 2007 and May 2008, found that one in five of them died.

Between January 2007 and December 2010, 2,329 children were admitted to Auckland's Starship Children's Hospital with a disease caused by *S. aureus*.[8] That's more than 10 a week. Of these, 163 children were classified as having a life-threatening invasive disease. In another study, in Gisborne in 2008, 110 children were diagnosed with a skin or soft tissue infection over a ten-week period.[9] On average, for every 14 children treated by their GP, one had to be hospitalised and would have required intravenous antibiotics, and perhaps even surgery. Findings from another study using hospital discharge data suggest that each year as many as 690 children under five may require hospitalisation for treatment of *S. aureus* skin and soft tissue infections, with almost 10 thousand more being treated by their GP.[10]

Compared with Pākehā children, four times as many Pasifika children and three times as many Māori children are hospitalised for serious skin infections. It's a similar story with adults, and with people living in our poorest households.

I'll delve later into why we have such high rates of *S. aureus* disease; for now, I'll just say that infectious microbes like *S. aureus* thrive when people don't have good access to healthcare or are living in overcrowded, cold or damp houses. It also doesn't help that the bacterium can be carried and spread by people without their realising it and that it can happily survive on inanimate objects in our homes, schools, workplaces, and hospitals. Hospitals have strict daily cleaning procedures to minimise the chances of patients picking up an infection. I'm not sure about you, but we don't have those same strict procedures in my house or where I work.

NEW ZEALAND'S SHAME
Streptococcus pyogenes is also known as strep or group A strep. When we microbiologists want to scare people, we call it the 'flesh-eating' bug, as it can sometimes digest human flesh, causing

necrotising fasciitis. This is a truly terrifying disease, which usually requires surgery to remove the infected flesh, and sometimes amputation to stop the bacteria from spreading throughout the body. It's fatal in about one of every five cases and can kill even very healthy young people.

Wellingtonian Rick Teal, a father of three in his thirties, had a near miss.[11] At work one day, one of his legs began to hurt. Two days later, doctors were removing large areas of flesh between his knee and ankle to save his life. Fit and healthy Royden Regler wasn't so lucky.[12] He died nine days after getting a hard knock to his thigh during a rugby match. No one realised his increasingly swollen leg was a case of necrotising fasciitis until too late. He was just twenty-three.

Almost everyone will have been infected with *S. pyogenes* at some stage in their life – it's a common cause of sore throats and tonsillitis. Many healthy people carry the bacterium in their throats without showing any symptoms – about one in a hundred adults and more than one in ten children. Like *S. aureus*, *S. pyogenes* can also cause a wide variety of illnesses, including skin and soft tissue infections, scarlet fever, bacteraemia, toxic shock syndrome, puerperal sepsis ('childbed fever'), and post-streptococcal glomerulonephritis, a rare complication that affects the kidneys.

Even a mild 'strep' throat can have lasting

consequences. Some people's bodies produce antibodies towards the bacterium that cross-react with the heart, joints, skin and brain, making them inflamed and swollen. This disease is called rheumatic fever. If the heart valves are damaged, it can lead to rheumatic heart disease, and surgery may be needed to replace the inflamed valves. To try to prevent rheumatic heart disease, people with rheumatic fever are usually given antibiotic injections every month for ten years or more.

Like *S. aureus*, *S. pyogenes* comes in hundreds of different varieties. This is one of the reasons why it has been difficult to develop an effective vaccine. A few years ago, the New Zealand and Australian Prime Ministers, John Key and Julia Gillard, pledged $3 million of joint funding to support the testing of three new vaccines.[13] The good news is that recent studies suggest that, if successful, one of the three would be able to protect us from about 60 to 70 per cent of the variants of *S. pyogenes* that cause disease in New Zealand.[14] The bad news is that $3 million is not a lot of money when it comes to vaccine development. It often takes more than ten years to deliver a licensed vaccine, at an estimated cost – from research and discovery to product registration – of $US500 million.[15] It's also been estimated that the probability of a pre-clinical vaccine reaching the market is about five to one against success.[16]

As with *S. aureus*, there have been attempts to calculate the burden of *S. pyogenes* disease in New Zealand, and it's the same grim story. Again, our rates are amongst the highest in the developed world and rising. Between 2002 and 2012, almost three thousand people – most of them under five or over seventy – were hospitalised with a serious *S. pyogenes* infection.[17] Again, Pasifika and Māori, as well as those living in our poorest households, were more likely to be affected. Another study found that the number of cases of necrotising fasciitis increased from ten a year in 1990 to seventy a year in 2006.[18] That was a decade ago. Has the number continued to rise since we last checked? It wouldn't surprise me.

But perhaps most shocking are our rates of rheumatic fever. A recent study found that they doubled between 2005 and 2010.[19] This disease mainly affects children between five and fourteen, and Māori and Pasifika children are twenty to forty times more likely to get it than other New Zealanders are. In fact, our rates are now among the highest in the world. In other words, hundreds of Kiwi kids each year are at risk of developing a life-threatening heart condition that is now extremely rare in other affluent countries like ours. It was brought under control in Europe and North America, experts believe, because of improvements in socioeconomic and housing conditions, combined with the use of antibiotics. To back this up, new research by Baker and his colleagues links our high rates to household crowding, financial deprivation, cold, damp homes, and living with smokers.[20]

A KICK IN THE GUTS

Around six in the evening of Friday 12 August 2016, the Hastings District Council began urging the residents of Havelock North to boil their water, and officials started chlorinating the town's water supply.[21] That day, thirteen people had presented to the emergency department of Hawke's Bay Regional Hospital with symptoms of a nasty gastrointestinal illness. By Monday, another sixty-eight people had gone to the emergency department, and 70 per cent of staff and students were absent from the town's schools. Havelock North had been struck by campylobacteriosis caused by *Campylobacter jejuni*, a helical-shaped bacterium commonly found in animal faeces.

People with campylobacteriosis can experience a week of cramping abdominal pain and watery or bloody diarrhoea, as well as fever, nausea and vomiting. For some, there can be long-term consequences, including Guillain–Barré syndrome (in which the immune system damages the nerves that join the spinal cord and brain to the rest of the body), reactive arthritis, and irritable bowel disease.

By the end of the outbreak – one of the largest ever in this country – an estimated 5,530 of Havelock North's residents had had symptoms of campylobacteriosis.[22] That's more than a third of the town's population. Forty-five ended up being hospitalised, and two elderly people died. Somehow the water supply had become contaminated with *C. jejuni*. Those bacteria were found to be of 'ruminant origin', according to the Institute of Environmental Science and Research (ESR).[23] Ruminant is another way of saying cattle, sheep and deer. The government launched an independent inquiry into the cause of the outbreak.[24]

Just as with *S. aureus* and *S. pyogenes*, our rates of campylobacteriosis are among the highest in the developed world. Even in a year without a Havelock North-sized outbreak, the disease affects thousands and hospitalises hundreds. In 2014, there were 6,776 cases across New Zealand, with 606 people admitted to hospital.[25] But *C. jejuni* isn't the only food- and water-borne microorganism that affects us. Joining it are organisms like *Giardia*, *Salmonella*, *Yersinia*, *Cryptosporidium*, toxin-producing *Escherichia coli*, rotavirus, norovirus, hepatitis A, *Leptospira*, and *Listeria*. Some of these organisms are found in our lakes and rivers; others live in the intestines of humans and animals.

Contact with farm animals is a major risk factor for catching many food- and water-borne infections.

No surprises then that farming regions served by the South Canterbury, West Coast, Waikato, Wairarapa and Northland district health boards (DHBs) are most affected. For similar geographical reasons, Pākehā have rates of disease two to three times higher than those of other New Zealanders. In 2014, food- and water-borne infections were responsible for 15,582 hospitalisations and 62 deaths.

In September of that year, New Zealand experienced one of the world's largest reported outbreaks of human yersiniosis caused by the bacterium *Yersinia pseudotuberculosis*.[26] There were 220 laboratory-confirmed cases, and 72 people were hospitalised. The source of the outbreak was never discovered; it was probably caused by people eating contaminated carrots and lettuce. But this is just the tip of the iceberg. Many more Kiwis will experience bouts of vomiting and diarrhoea that go unrecorded.

ONE LAST HIDDEN DANGER

There's another microorganism we need to start taking more notice of, even though it doesn't really feature in the hospitalisation records. *Chlamydia trachomatis* is a bacterium that can be transmitted from person to person during vaginal, anal and oral sex. It can also be passed from an infected mother to her baby during childbirth. In babies, infection can lead to blindness and pneumonia.

The symptoms of chlamydia in women include abnormal vaginal discharge, bleeding between periods, pain when having sex or peeing, and an itching or burning in or around the genitals. In men, it's pain when peeing, pain and swelling around the testicles, a clear or cloudy discharge from the tip of the penis, and a burning and itching around the penis opening. The good news is that chlamydia is still easily treated with antibiotics, and even better, it's preventable by using condoms and dental dams during sex.

Chlamydia isn't a notifiable disease in New Zealand, so doctors don't have to report how many cases they see to the Ministry of Health. The best estimates put our rate at 629 cases per 100,000 population, which is the way public health people describe these things.[27] Yet again, we are topping the charts; our rates are double those of Australia and the UK. Rates range from about 330 cases per 100,000 for the West Coast DHB region, to about 1,140 for the Lakes DHB.

So why are our rates so high? In a recent survey, fewer than half of sexually active young people reported using condoms. Learning about sexually transmitted infections is part of sexuality education in the curriculum. But schools can choose to leave it out, or parents can opt to remove their children from class.

I wonder if part of the wider problem is the

shame we seem to associate with sex and women's genitalia. A few years ago, a British gynaecological cancer charity, the Eve Appeal, found that two-thirds of young women it surveyed had a problem using the words vagina or vulva, and nearly 40 per cent said they use euphemisms instead – terms like 'lady parts', 'bits', 'front bottom' and 'vajayjay'. When we use such phrases, we stigmatise these essential parts of our body. Like something we need to hide. Even worse, the Eve Appeal found that many young women couldn't correctly identify their internal and external genitalia on a simple diagram. Do you know a vagina from a vulva, or where the cervix and labia are? If yes, great. If not, why not?

For me, what makes chlamydia scary is that seven out of ten infected women, and one in every four infected men, will have no symptoms at all. *C. trachomatis* will be happily living inside people who remain unaware they are infected. This really matters, because, without antibiotic treatment, about half of asymptomatic women will go on to develop pelvic inflammatory disease – a generic term for infection of the uterus, fallopian tubes, ovaries, and surrounding tissues.

Pelvic inflammatory disease can scar and permanently damage the reproductive organs, causing serious complications like chronic pelvic pain, ectopic pregnancy and infertility. It's a similar story for asymptomatic men. If untreated, they can develop painful swelling of the testicles and epididymis (that's the tube located at the back of the testicles that stores and carries sperm), as well as reactive arthritis and infertility.

Let's do some back-of-the-envelope calculations. According to the most recent publicly available figures, in 2014 there were 28,331 cases of lab-confirmed chlamydia. Of those, 19,986 were in women. If this represents the roughly three in ten with symptoms of infection, there could be a staggering 46,634 women and young girls with asymptomatic chlamydia at risk of disease and infertility later in life. For the men and young boys, it works out to 24,825 at risk.

Infertility is a serious issue. It's heart-breaking for the couples involved, and a massive threat to the future prosperity of our country. A falling birth rate and an ageing population are not a good combination. Yes, science can help with techniques like in vitro fertilisation (IVF), but that's an emotionally and physically demanding, and financially expensive, solution to a preventable problem.

C. trachomatis is not the only microorganism that threatens our sexual health. Later in this book, I'll introduce you to another infectious microbe and yet more reasons for getting our sexually transmitted infections under control.

3. A NEW ERA OF MEDICINE DAWNS

Now that you have met some of our bacterial foes, it's time to meet the medicines used to treat the infections they cause. Maybe it's because I'm a medical researcher, but whenever a doctor prescribes my family or me medication, I wonder where it comes from. I don't mean where it was physically made (I'll touch on that later), but how it came into being. I start to think about all the people and their experiments that led to its approval as a medicine. What was their eureka moment?

Professor Paul Ehrlich (1854–1915) was a German physician and scientist who was a pioneer in the field of using dyes to stain tissue samples for examination under a microscope. When he began his career in the 1880s, infectious diseases were the leading cause of death in Europe. Life expectancy in Germany was under forty. When

Ehrlich discovered that some dyes were able to stain microorganisms, he wondered whether they could also interfere with them in some way and so be used to kill them during an infection. The first dye he tried – methylene blue – reduced the fever of two patients with malaria, an infectious disease caused by the parasite *Plasmodium*.

Convinced he was onto something, Ehrlich turned his lab to the task of testing hundreds of chemicals for antimicrobial activity. In 1909, his assistant Dr Sahachiro Hata (1873–1938) found that 'compound 606' (arsphenamine) killed the bacteria that cause syphilis, *Treponema*. In 1910, the chemical company Hoechst AG began to manufacture arsphenamine and market it for treating syphilis under the name Salvarsan. The drug quickly became very popular. Syphilis was rampant in Europe at the time, and Salvarsan was more effective and much safer than the previous treatment, mercury salts. Even so, it was hard to store and prepare, and not without its side-effects.

Professor Gerhard Domagk (1895–1964) was another German physician and scientist interested in infectious diseases. In the late 1890s he was appointed the director of Bayer's Institute of Pathology and Bacteriology, where he worked on Ehrlich's idea of using dyes as antimicrobials. At the time, Germany's chemical industry dominated the world market for synthetic dyes and was keen to expand into other areas, including the search for medicines. In 1925, Bayer merged with Hoechst AG and four other German chemical companies to form IG Farben. The merger gave Domagk access to thousands of synthetic dyes and related compounds to test.

In the early 1930s he discovered that a red dye called sulphonamidochrysoidine was able to protect mice against infection with the 'flesh-eating' bacteria we met earlier, *S. pyogenes*. Marketed as Prontosil, the drug was soon being used to successfully treat infections like puerperal sepsis, which killed many women shortly after childbirth (often because their babies had been delivered by doctors who had just been working on cadavers in the morgue and hadn't washed their hands between the two activities).

Prontosil was the first medicine ever discovered that could be effectively used to treat several different bacterial infections inside the body. Interestingly, it has no effect on bacteria in the lab.

Sulphonamidochrysoidine is what is known as a prodrug. These are drugs that our bodies metabolise into the active compound. It turned out that the active compound, sulphanilamide, was already widely used in the dye-making industry and had been patented in 1909. Because its patent had already expired, anyone was now able to make the drug. This spurred chemists around the world to create thousands of patentable sulphanilamide derivatives, known as sulphonamides.

Many sulphonamides were found to have antibacterial activity (although they are bacteriostatic meaning they don't kill bacteria but stop them multiplying), and they are credited with saving many lives, including Winston Churchill's. During the Second World War, American soldiers were issued with a first-aid kit containing a sulphonamide powder for sprinkling on open wounds.

As well as providing a class of antibiotics, some sulphonamides were active against viruses, while others are now used to treat diabetes, high blood pressure, seizures and arthritis.

The testing of synthetic chemicals in the 1950s and 60s also led to the development of other classes of antibiotics that work in different ways, including fluoroquinolones and nitroimidazoles. Some of these drugs are still used to treat people today.

THE ANTIMICROBIAL 'GOLD RUSH'

While the Germans were methodically testing thousands of dyes, a Scottish scientist working at St Mary's Hospital in London was rediscovering the antibiotic properties of microorganisms themselves.[1] Dr Alexander Fleming (1881–1955) was studying staphylococci, the family of bacteria that includes *S. aureus*. In September 1928, he returned to work after a holiday to find one of his cultures contaminated with a fungus. This often happens to us microbiologists because so many fungal spores float around in the air!

In Fleming's case, though, the fungi had killed all the bacterial colonies it touched. He grew the fungus and discovered that it produced a substance that could kill *S. aureus*, *S. pyogenes*, and some other disease-causing bacteria. He identified the fungus as a species of *Penicillium* and published his findings in the June 1929 issue of the *British Journal of Experimental Pathology*.[2]

In his paper, Fleming named the antibacterial substance penicillin 'for convenience and to avoid the repetition of the rather cumbersome phrase "Mould broth filtrate"'. He suggested it would make an 'efficient antiseptic' for treating some infections and would be useful to microbiologists trying to culture bacteria that were often outcompeted by faster-growing or more abundant species. We now know that penicillin is a beta-lactam antibiotic that stops some bacteria building their cell walls, causing them to die.

Throughout the 1930s, Fleming continued to work on penicillin but found the antibiotic difficult to produce in large quantities. It took a team working at the University of Oxford, led by Australian Professor Howard Florey (1898–1968), to make penicillin the wonder drug it became.

Together with Dr Ernst Chain (1906–1979) and Dr Norman Heatley (1911–2004), Florey turned his lab into the first penicillin factory and showed that the antibiotic could be used to treat infections in mice and people.

But they still struggled to produce penicillin in sufficient amounts, so in 1941 Florey and Heatley travelled to the United States to try to interest others in mass-producing it. Scientists at the Northern Regional Research Laboratory in Illinois took up the challenge, and by 1945, after a worldwide search for a better strain of *Penicillium*, billions of units of penicillin were being produced to treat wounded Allied soldiers.

The success of penicillin sparked the antimicrobial equivalent of a gold rush. Scientists from academic and industry labs around the world started testing for antimicrobial compounds. They looked at thousands of microorganisms isolated from soils, compost and peats. I read somewhere that the US Army Transport Corps was contracted to collect soil samples from wherever its planes landed!

With all this research going on, the 1940s and 50s were a hugely productive time for antibiotic discovery. Almost all of the classes of antibiotics we use today date from this period: the aminoglycosides, ansamycins, chloramphenicols, glycopeptides, lipopeptides, macrolides, oxazolidinones, polymyxins, streptogramins and tetracyclines. All are based on compounds made by microorganisms.

But the hunt for new antibiotics became a game of diminishing returns. Time and time again, the same ones were 'rediscovered'. Between the 1960s and 80s, just three new antibiotic classes were discovered from microbial sources: carbapenems, lincosamides and monobactams. It was clearly time for a new strategy.

THE ERA OF 'TARGETED' ANTIBIOTIC DESIGN

Producing and purifying antibiotics from environmental bacteria and fungi is not an easy task. Efforts quickly turned to deciphering each antibiotic's chemical structure and figuring out how they all worked. This paved the way for antibiotics to be chemically synthesised rather than harnessed from the original microbial source, making the whole endeavour more efficient and safer. It also allowed chemists to develop better derivatives of existing antibiotics by tweaking their chemical structures.

But this also led to a rise in 'me-too' antibiotics, drugs from the same class developed by competing companies. By the 1980s, instead of producing an array of novel compounds, the antibiotic discovery pipeline had become less innovative and was delivering fewer new drugs over time. It's easy to see why no one was concerned. Antibiotics had ushered in a new era of medicine, enabling the development of many life-saving medical procedures. People in Europe and the US were now living into their seventies, and cardiovascular diseases, cancer and neurological conditions had replaced infectious diseases as the leading causes of death.

By the 1990s, microbiology as a scientific discipline was undergoing a revolution. The genomic era was well under way, and scientists were developing new 'molecular' techniques to engineer bacteria genetically. Now, microbiologists could insert or disrupt specific genes within the particular bacterium they were interested in, and find out which genes different bacteria use for causing disease, and which are needed by the bacteria to grow and survive.

This, and the sequencing of the first bacterial genome (in other words, all of a bacteria's genetic material) in the mid-1990s, signalled a new phase of antibiotic discovery. Out went the traditional approach of testing chemicals against living bacterial cells and seeing if they survived or died. Now, each bacteria's genetic code could be used to identify specific 'targets' that researchers could develop specific drugs to inhibit. This was targeted drug design.

While the approach was a great success in the development of antivirals for treating HIV, it failed spectacularly for developing new antibiotics.

Despite thirty-four companies chasing sixty different bacterial targets, not a single credible antibacterial candidate was deemed suitable for further development.[3]

The pharmaceutical industry has now largely pulled out of antibiotic research and the pipeline has more or less shut down. There are just three new antibiotics going through clinical trials that are listed as 'high priority', meaning they could potentially be used against resistant superbugs.[4]

As a general rule, only one in five compounds for treating infectious diseases that enter phase 1 clinical trials end up being approved for use in patients. In the next chapter, I'll explain why this is something that should make us all very anxious.

4. ANTIMICROBIAL RESISTANCE

A common misconception I hear when talking to people about antimicrobial resistance is that it's us who become resistant to the drugs. This is a reason people give for trying to avoid using antibiotics so that the antibiotics will work for them when they need them. But the correct definition of antimicrobial resistance is the ability of microorganisms to grow in the presence of a particular antimicrobial compound. In other words, it's the microorganisms that are resistant, not us.

Some microorganisms are intrinsically resistant to the effects of particular classes of antimicrobial compounds; others develop resistance, and the agents that once killed them or stopped them from growing lose their power. It's this development of resistance that has health experts worried.

Actually, that's putting it mildly. Terrified is probably more like it. Previously treatable microorganisms are becoming untreatable. This means that previously treatable infections will once again become deadly, or may require amputation to stop them in their tracks. And because antimicrobials are also used to prevent infection in vulnerable people, it will also become life-threateningly risky to do routine operations like caesarean sections and joint replacements, or use treatments like chemotherapy for cancer.

The head of the World Health Organization (WHO), Margaret Chan, has called antimicrobial resistance 'the end of modern medicine as we know it'.[1] In a series of reports commissioned by then British Prime Minister David Cameron, economist Lord O'Neill has estimated that without urgent action, antimicrobial resistance will kill 10 million people a year by 2050 – more than will die from cancer.[2]

THE 'HOW' OF ANTIMICROBIAL RESISTANCE

How resistance happens depends on the particular microorganism and antimicrobial compound. For example, some bacteria have developed ways to stop certain antibiotics from getting inside them, or use pumps to push others back out before they take effect. Other bacteria produce destructive enzymes to neutralise particular antibiotics. Bacteria can also modify an antibiotic's target (the bit of them that the antibiotic acts on) so that the antibiotic is no longer effective. Alternatively, they can create bypasses that allow them to function even when the antibiotic's target is being inhibited.

If all this sounds like bacteria are actively conspiring against antibiotics, they're not. Rather, resistance is a natural result of a normal process that goes on in all our cells every day. It's the process by which even we adapt and evolve to our surroundings.

As a cell replicates its genetic material, there is a chance it will make some mistakes. Most of these errors are picked up by the cell's repair systems, but a small number can make it into the newly produced cell. We call these mutations. Their effect varies according to where they are. A mutation might change the expression of a particular gene, or create a mutant protein – or it might make no difference at all. If the mutation gives the bacteria an advantage, then it can outgrow the other bacteria and become the dominant or only strain that remains. This is known as selection.

To put this in perspective, let's take *S. aureus*, which causes all those skin and soft tissue infections in children. Under ideal conditions in the lab, it can replicate itself about every half-hour. This means that a single *S. aureus* cell can grow into a population of more than a million in 12 hours and a billion in 15. That's a billion opportunities for mistakes to be made and mutations to slip through. If any of those mutations confer an advantage or at least don't put the bacterium at a disadvantage, they will be the ones that survive. In other words, antibiotic resistance can emerge purely by chance as bacteria grow.

Resistance to some antibiotics requires a very specific mutation or one of a handful of mutations. For others, it needs more than one mutation. Some genes are also more prone to mutations than others – and here is where it gets scarier. If bacteria are exposed to an inadequate antibiotic dose, instead of quickly killing them all, the antibiotic puts them under stress so that they make more mutations, thus boosting the chance of their becoming resistant. This can happen wherever bacteria encounter antibiotics, whether that's within a patient or out in the environment. I'll explain more about that later.

THE MOBILE NATURE OF RESISTANCE

Although the antibiotic resistance that emerges by mutation and is passed on by a bacterium to its descendants is worrying, it is limited to that particular bacterial strain. But bacteria can take resistance to another level, thanks to what we call horizontal gene transfer.

Genetic material can move not only between different cells of the same species but between cells of entirely different species. It does this by various means, including via plasmids – extra, smaller bits of genetic material outside the organism's chromosome – and transposons, which are like jumping tweezers moving in and out of chromosomes and plasmids, plucking up and depositing bits of genetic material as they go. Some bacteria can take up genetic material, including plasmids, from their environment through a process known as *transformation*. Bacteria can also exchange plasmids (sometimes forcibly) in a process called *conjugation*. This requires the bacteria to be in direct contact, so the plasmids can arrange for the bacteria to build the equivalent of a bridge between them.

Finally, genetic material can also move between bacteria via viruses known as bacteriophage (phage for short). As I explained earlier, viruses rely on the machinery of the cell they've infected to replicate their genetic material. When a virus infects a bacterium, it can accidentally incorporate genetic material from its host's plasmids or chromosome as it replicates and makes new viruses. These in turn can transfer that material into their next host cell. This process is known as *transduction*.

Transduction, conjugation and transformation have all contributed to the widespread dissemination of antibiotic resistance, even into bacterial species that have never even encountered the antibiotics they are now resistant to. In environments around the world – soil, water, faeces – bacteria are moving antibiotic resistance genes around.

To summarise: bacteria can be naturally resistant to antibiotics or can develop resistance by mutating or acquiring resistance genes from another bacterium. What that means is that you don't even have to have taken an antibiotic to have resistant bacteria living inside you right now. Now we'll move on to why that might be the case.

THE POWER OF SELECTION, OR, WHY RESISTANCE HAPPENS

As noted already in this chapter, antimicrobial resistance is natural and inevitable. Evolving and adapting is what life does, and bacteria do it very rapidly. If you want to watch antibiotic resistance happen right in front of your eyes, a microbiologist at Harvard Medical School, Dr Michael Baym, has captured it on video. You can watch online at https://vimeo.com/180908160.

Baym came up with an ingenious experiment to show resistance in action. He and his colleagues developed a giant Petri dish, more than half a metre wide and a metre long, divided into sections. The outermost sections contain no antibiotic, just the jelly (called agar) on which bacteria like to grow. The next sections in contain a little bit of an antibiotic called trimethoprim that a lab strain of

E. coli can survive in. The next sections in contain ten times more trimethoprim than *E. coli* can typically withstand; and the final section in the middle contains a thousand times more. On top of all this agar, Baym adds another thinner layer of agar that *E. coli* can swim through. Then he adds *E. coli* to the outer sections, turns on the time-lapse camera, and waits.

The results are mesmerising. First, the bacteria grow all over the outermost segments, until they reach the first concentration of antibiotic. Mutants emerge that then grow and spread until they reach the next concentration. The same thing happens again and again until, after just eleven days, mutants of *E. coli* have evolved that can grow at a thousand times the concentration of trimethoprim that would have killed them.

Baym has done this for lots of different antibiotics, and even disinfectants that the manufacturers claim the bacteria can't become resistant to. They do.

Not only do Baym's experiments show how quickly antimicrobial resistance can emerge, they beautifully illustrate the power of selection: mutants survive when they have an advantage. And what better way to have an advantage than when antimicrobials are present? In other words, antimicrobial use *drives* resistance.

Would you be surprised if I told you that

antibiotic resistance has existed for thousands, if not millions, of years?[3] It has, but not to the extent that it does now. Humans aren't the only ones who exploit antibiotics. Remember how penicillin was discovered from a fungus? Given the microbial origin of most antibiotics, it's more than likely they are also utilised by bacteria and fungi fighting for space and nutrients in their natural habitats. But this pales in comparison with our use and misuse of antibiotics. In the next chapter, I'll explore this and the antibiotic-resistant 'superbugs' that have arisen as a result.

5. HOW ANTIBIOTICS ARE USED

The Center for Disease Dynamics, Economics, and Policy (CDDEP) is a public health research organisation with headquarters in the United States and India. According to its 2015 report on the global use of antibiotics (a report, by the way, that excludes Australia and New Zealand 'because of data reliability issues') the quantity of antibiotics used in human medicine around the world increased from 50 billion to 70 billion standard units (SU) between 2000 and 2010.[1] This measure is broadly based on the smallest dose given to a patient; think of one SU as the equivalent of one antibiotic pill or capsule. So, in 2010, humans used the equivalent of at least 70 billion antibiotic pills.

But it's not infectious diseases that are behind the antibiotic boom – it's the economic growth of the rapidly growing countries known as the BRICS

(Brazil, Russia, India, China and South Africa). Despite accounting for only a third of the world's population increase between 2000 and 2010, these five countries accounted for three-quarters of the increase in antibiotic use. In 2010, the top users were India with 13 billion SU, China (10 billion), and the US (7 billion). When we take population size into account, the US comes out on top, with twenty-two SU per person, double India's rate and three times China's.

The CDDEP also estimates that 80 per cent of our medical use of antibiotics happens outside hospitals. While some of this will be antibiotics being prescribed by clinics and GPs' surgeries, it also includes people taking them without a prescription. There are two main sources of unprescribed antibiotics: pharmacies, and friends and family. By law, in most countries at least, some antibiotics are only available on prescription. But it turns out these laws aren't enforced in most low- and middle-income countries and some high-income countries. For example, a 2010 study of pharmacies in Vietnam found that nine out of ten antibiotic sales were without a prescription. In Saudi Arabia, a study showed it was about eight out of ten.

If antibiotics aren't being prescribed by a qualified health professional, the big question is: are they being used in the right way? The answer is: probably not. In fact, it's thought that up to half of all antibiotics used medically might fall into this category. In other words, they are being misused.

There are two main ways this can happen. The first is taking them to treat diseases that they won't help. This includes diseases not caused by bacteria, like malaria and influenza, or bacterial infections that will clear up without antibiotics, like some forms of food poisoning. The second is when they are used 'sub-optimally' – for example, by taking too low a dose for it to be properly effective or using an antibiotic that kills lots of different kinds of bacteria (so-called 'broad-spectrum') instead of one that is more specific ('narrow-spectrum').

Broad-spectrum antibiotics are often prescribed because they don't taste as bad, or can be taken with food, or require fewer doses each day. But these are usually not good enough reasons for using them when a narrow-spectrum alternative is available. Another sub-optimal use is stopping a course of antibiotics too soon, perhaps because of side-effects, or because your symptoms have cleared up and you want to save the rest of the bottle for future use.

A little later, I'll explain how the misuse of antibiotics has contributed to growing global disasters that have already touched our shores and will do so again. But here's a simple example of personal misuse: let's say someone has diarrhoea/a sore throat/fever and takes a broad-spectrum antibiotic until their condition clears up a few days later. What they've just done is the equivalent of burning down a forest to get rid of one tree. They've wiped out many beneficial bacteria and given antibiotic-resistant strains the opportunity to evolve and dominate.

In cases like these, the antibiotic-resistant bacteria don't make you ill. They just live on or inside you and spread to others in your community. And then one day, maybe a week later, maybe ten years later, they do give someone diarrhoea/a sore throat/fever – only this time the antibiotics don't work. Depending on the microorganism, this can mean a personal tragedy or a full-scale public health disaster.

Before you go thinking this just happens in low- and middle-income countries, a study involving six US hospitals in 2009 and 2010 found that a third of the patients prescribed antibiotics for an infection had no clinical signs of infection. And nearly two-thirds of the patients who *did* have symptoms were left on antibiotics even when their tests came back clear!

Many low- and middle-income countries are guilty of using antibiotics as a cheap alternative to preventing infection in the first place. Strengthening hygiene and infection control in hospitals, providing sanitation, and improving access to clean water and vaccines are all relatively expensive, way more so than antibiotics, most of which are off-patent and cheap and easy to manufacture.

ANTIBIOTICS AND ANIMALS

Before going more deeply into industrial antibiotic use, I want to touch briefly on antibiotic use in our pets. Just as in humans, antibiotic misuse applies to our pets, too. Because of how physically close we often get to them, they can be an overlooked source of both antibiotic-sensitive and antibiotic-resistant bacteria, including *S. aureus* and *E. coli*. And vice-versa!

The use of antibiotics in pets pales in comparison, however, with their use in production animals. Reliable information isn't widely available but data from countries that do record such use suggests that it's at least as high as the amount used by humans, and probably higher. For example, in 2010 the US Food and Drug Administration (FDA) reported that more than 70 per cent of all US sales of medically important antibiotics were for use in animals.

It's estimated that between 63,000 and 240,000 tonnes of antibiotics are being used globally in agriculture.[2] And this is projected to rise as the BRICS's economic growth drives the demand for more meat and dairy products. The CDDEP estimates that this demand will increase global antibiotic use in agriculture by almost 70 per cent between 2010 and 2030.[3] In 2010, China was estimated to be the highest user, followed by the US, Brazil, Germany and India. Modelling by CDDEP researchers suggests that the pattern will be similar in 2030, but with Mexico replacing Germany in the top five.

Antibiotics have been used to prevent or treat infections in animals for almost as long as we've been using them to treat people, and most of the ones used in agriculture are similar to those used in people. The top three classes by global sales (macrolides, penicillins and tetracyclines) are all categorised by the WHO as critically important for human medicine.

But antibiotics have another use in agriculture. In 1950, scientists in the US discovered quite by accident that the antibiotic aureomycin had a remarkable effect on poultry. When fed to birds and animals in low doses, it made them grow and reach their full market weight much faster. Farmers were soon using antibiotics as so-called 'growth promoters'.

From what you've learned about the development and selection of resistance so far in this book, I'm sure you'll agree that the use of antibiotics as growth promoters is not a good idea. The European Union agrees; it banned this type of use in 2006. According to reports on the subject, Australia has a partial ban, whereas it's voluntary in the US. As for much of the rest of the world, we don't have the data to know.

I must admit that I think the debate over antibiotics as growth promoters is a bit of a red herring. By far their biggest use in agriculture is to prevent infection. We've known for a long time that overcrowding and poor sanitation lead to outbreaks of infectious diseases. This applies to animals as well as to humans, but the intensification of agriculture in recent decades has brought large numbers of animals into closer and closer proximity. Because of this, antibiotics and other antimicrobials are widely used to keep animals healthy and maintain production, and to stop diseases from sweeping through flocks and herds.

Just as with use in humans, the relatively low cost of these products makes them cheaper than vaccinating, improving sanitation, and farming less intensively. So, while intensive agriculture has reduced the price of food, it has likely done so at the far greater cost of contributing to antimicrobial resistance. And with growing demand for meat and dairy products around the world, this type of antibiotic use is only going to increase.

ANTIBIOTICS AND THE ENVIRONMENT

Most of the antibiotics we and our animals ingest aren't broken down, but pass through the body and into our faeces, ending up in wastewater treatment plants and in the soil and water. So we're not only breeding antibiotic-resistant bacteria in our bodies and the bodies of our animals, we're helping antibiotic-resistant bacteria to survive in the wider environment too.

But this isn't the only way antibiotics and other antimicrobials get into the environment. Take aquaculture – a booming industry around the globe. Most of the world's shrimp and carnivorous fish are produced in Asia, so aquaculture accounts for a large share of the antibiotic use in an increasing number of countries in South-East Asia. Similarly, Chile is a major producer of farmed salmon, which are raised using at least a dozen antibiotics.[4] The CDDEP report warns that as the aquaculture industry grows and shifts toward more 'efficient' (that is, intensive) production systems, it could become a major source of antimicrobial contamination of our water.

It doesn't have to be that way. With strict regulation, the use of antibiotics in aquaculture in Norway fell by 99 per cent between 1987 and 2013. By using vaccines, and with better farm hygiene and management, the industry's output grew by nearly 2,000 per cent over the same time.

It's estimated that less than half a per cent of all the antibiotics used in agriculture go on crops. Before saying more about this, I want to tell you about a meeting I had with representatives of Zespri during the Psa outbreak. In 2010, this bacterium (Psa is short for *Pseudomonas syringae* pv. *actinidiae*) threatened to destroy New Zealand's kiwifruit industry, and Zespri was consulting widely with the scientific community about what to do. At the meeting, someone from the company asked what antibiotics they could spray all the vines with to kill Psa. My colleagues and I were horrified. Psa is from the same family as *P. aeruginosa*, which can cause a range of infections in vulnerable people, including those with the inherited disease cystic fibrosis. All we could think of was antibiotic-resistant Psa developing, and transferring resistance to bacteria like *P. aeruginosa*, which would kill people. All to save our kiwifruit industry.

We explained the problem with that idea, and the subject was dropped, but it was a stark example of the lack of communication between people working in human medicine and in agriculture/aquaculture. This is one reason why there are moves around the world, and in New Zealand, to adopt a 'One Health' approach to infectious diseases. It's clear that the health of humans, animals, plants and the environment are all inextricably linked. 'One Health' initiatives bring together people working on infectious microbes in all these different areas to share knowledge and raise understanding.

Back to crop plants. Anyone who loves gardening will know that plants frequently battle fungal diseases. The same goes for crops. In the late 1990s, doctors in the Netherlands started to see patients suffering from severe disease caused by strains of the fungus *Aspergillus fumigatus* that were resistant to a class of antifungal medicines called azoles. It turns out that this is because in the Netherlands it's standard practice to dip every tulip bulb in fungicide before it's planted.

But the Netherlands is not the only place that uses azoles. Britain's Review on Antimicrobial Resistance chaired by Lord O'Neill found that almost half of European cereals and grapevines are treated at least once a year, compared with less than 5 per cent in the US. Europe's wetter climate and different soil may explain this difference. *A. fumigatus* is naturally found in the soil, so even though the same azoles aren't used in agriculture and human medicine, the resistance mutations are. This means that the use of azoles in the agricultural sector has driven the development of resistant strains that can cause untreatable disease in people.

A. fumigatus is a particular problem for patients with weakened immune systems, and azole-based medicines are crucial for fighting these. Azole-resistant strains of *A. fumigatus* have now been reported all over Europe, as well as throughout the rest of the world.[5] More than half of patients with an invasive azole-resistant *A. fumigatus* infection die.

Another way antibiotics end up in our environment is the waste from the factories where they are manufactured. A recent report on the subject by the European Public Health Alliance (EPHA) makes grim reading.[6] According to the report, most of the world's drugs are made by contract manufacturers in China and India, but the supply chain is 'complex and opaque'. It's believed that 80 to 90 per cent of the active ingredients needed to make antibiotics are manufactured in China, while India has positioned itself as a cost-effective place to make the finished products.

In 2006, Swedish scientists studied effluent samples from a wastewater treatment plant near Hyderabad in India.[7] At the time, the plant was taking 1.5 million litres of wastewater a day, trucked in from about ninety different drug manufacturers that were either synthesising active ingredients or making finished products. After treatment, the wastewater was discharged into a stream feeding several rivers. The scientists found that the samples contained by far the highest levels of pharmaceuticals ever reported in any effluent, including high levels of several broad-spectrum antibiotics.

There is no reason to think things have improved in the past decade. The EPHA report lists recent instances of Chinese and Indian companies illegally dumping their waste into rivers and onto nearby land or burying it in secret pits. These are companies with links to major international pharmaceutical companies you'd recognise from seeing their products advertised on TV – GlaxoSmithKline, Wyeth, Novartis, Pfizer, Sanofi, Roche.

The main problem is that regulators like the UK's Medicines and Healthcare Products Regulatory Authority, the European Medicines Agency, and the FDA, which license companies to make drugs for their markets, only require manufacturers to meet a set of safety standards that don't cover environmental emissions.

What about New Zealand's Pharmaceutical Management Agency (Pharmac), which sources our antibiotics? Do their standards cover environmental emissions? I can't find any mention of it on their website.

In 2016, thirteen pharmaceutical companies pledged to review their manufacturing and supply chains and reduce the impact of their wastewater discharges by 2020.[8] I don't think a pledge is good enough. And by 2020?! No. An issue as crucial as this needs independent oversight now, and massive financial penalties for companies that don't behave responsibly.

6. ANTIBIOTIC USE IN NEW ZEALAND

So how does New Zealand fare for antibiotic use? When the New Zealand Veterinary Association's (NZVA) Strategic Group on Antimicrobial Resistance analysed data from official government and industry reports for New Zealand, Australia, Canada, Britain, the US and twenty-six European countries in 2014, New Zealand came out the third lowest user of antimicrobials in food production.[1] The NZVA did the review because it has set a vision that by 2030 'New Zealand Inc will not need antibiotics for the maintenance of animal health and wellness'.

In New Zealand, antibiotics are classed as restricted veterinary medicines and agricultural chemicals. The Ministry for Primary Industries (MPI) analyses sales to provide information about their use in food production. The sales data doesn't necessarily equate to actual use, but MPI interprets it in consultation with vets and other people from the various food production industries. The most recent sales report (October 2016) covers the years 2011–14.[2]

But before we have a look at what it says, I want to dig a little deeper into that statistic about New Zealand being the third lowest user of antimicrobials in food production. One of the main reasons is that we farm our cattle and sheep – the bulk of our production animals by weight – almost exclusively out on pasture. In other countries, this is not usually the case. For example, beef cattle in the US, Brazil and Argentina are 'finished' in large feedlots where they are given antibiotics. So what do we use antibiotics for in food production then?

Back to that MPI report. The first finding from the data is that sales rose between 2011 and 2014, particularly to the horticultural industry, which the report puts down to managing the kiwifruit Psa outbreak with streptomycin and kasugamycin. Turns out antibiotics were used after all!

Kasugamycin is not used in human medicine but has been used in horticulture in some countries since the 1960s, mainly to control some diseases of rice, apples and pears. Bacteria resistant to kasugamycin have been reported overseas,[3] but fortunately the resistance they have evolved doesn't make them resistant to other similar antibiotics that are used in humans.

Streptomycin on the other hand is used in human medicine, sometimes as part of a cocktail of drugs to treat tuberculosis but also for the plague, as well as for urinary tract infections and pneumonia caused by bacteria resistant to safer antibiotics. Plasmid-based resistance to streptomycin has been reported overseas, so we should be cautious.

Saying that, even with the Psa outbreak, antibiotic sales to the horticultural industry only accounted for less than 2 per cent of the total – as did sales for pets. While the amount used is small, some of the antibiotics sold are listed as 'critically important' for human health. As I've explained earlier, our pets can be a source of both antibiotic-sensitive and antibiotic-resistant bacteria.

The vast majority of antibiotics sold for use in animals in New Zealand are for cattle, pigs and poultry. The number of pigs farmed here is declining as more and more pork is imported, so the rise in antibiotic sales recorded in the MPI report can probably be attributed to greater numbers of poultry and dairy cattle. The number of chickens bred for meat went up by 11 per cent from 93 million in 2011 to 103 million in 2014. Just 15 million of these were free-range; the rest were reared in barns. The number of egg-laying hens also rose, from 3.5 million to almost 4 million over the same period. Fewer than half a million of our layers are free-range; the rest are caged.

According to the report, half of the antibiotics sold between 2011 and 2014 were for administering to poultry and pigs via food, so it's likely these are being used to prevent infection. Similarly, antibiotics are widely used in the dairy industry to treat and prevent mastitis. This category accounted for about 15 per cent of antibiotics sales. The national dairy herd grew to 4.9 million in 2013–14, when the average herd size was 413, up from 386 in 2011–12. As the report notes, the larger the herd, the greater the risk of disease and cross-contamination. In fact, the average herd size has since grown to 419 in 2015–16.

To summarise, while our use of antibiotics in food production is low compared to other countries, that's more because the majority of our large animals are raised outside on grass. But most of our poultry are intensively farmed and fed antibiotics. Whether that's to prevent infection or promote growth, the outcome is the same. Between 2011 and 2014, there were increased sales in New Zealand of four classes of antibiotics classified as critically important to human medicine. These increases ranged from 18 to 55 per cent. That is nothing to be proud of.

ANTIBIOTIC USE IN PEOPLE IN NEW ZEALAND

Information about all drugs used in human medicine and subsidised by the government is held by the Ministry of Health and Pharmac in a data 'warehouse' called the Pharmaceutical Collection. Deborah Williamson and colleagues looked at the data for 'antibacterials' for the years 2006–14.[4] For some reason, this category doesn't include information on antibiotic-containing creams or antibiotics used to treat TB. Nevertheless, the findings show that antibiotic use in New Zealand has risen rapidly and is high by international standards.

Williamson and her colleagues discovered that about 36 million prescriptions were made out for antibiotics between 2006 and 2014. Over that time, antibiotic use in New Zealand increased by almost 50 per cent! Compared with other OECD and some other European countries, including Australia, Britain and Canada, our use is high. We rank in the top third, beaten only by Romania, France, Italy, Korea, Belgium and Luxembourg.

In Chapter 2, I explained that we have high rates of many infectious diseases, but the prescribing data suggests that this is not the whole reason why our antibiotic use is so high. For starters, it doesn't include the antibiotic-containing creams used to treat *S. aureus* skin and soft tissue infections. Instead the data shows that antibiotic use varies throughout the year, peaking in the winter months. This suggests that a large proportion may be being prescribed for seasonal conditions such as viral infections. (Remember, antibiotics don't work against viruses.)

Amoxicillin with clavulanate is also quite heavily used in New Zealand. According to Williamson and her colleagues, there are very few infections for which this combination of antibiotics is the 'first-line' choice, which suggests it may be being used in the wrong way.

The data shows that antibiotic use in New Zealand is highest in the elderly and young children, which isn't surprising, given that these are the people most at risk of getting many infections. In terms of ethnicity, use is highest among Pasifika. While this does reflect their high burden of infectious diseases, it could also indicate cultural differences in knowledge or understanding of antibiotics.

Professor Pauline Norris focuses her research on access to, and use of, medicines.[5] She and her Otago University colleagues have looked into antibiotic use by people of different ethnicities. In one of their studies, they surveyed people of Samoan descent living in New Zealand.[6] They found that only a few knew what antibiotics were for; two-thirds thought they were for pain relief, like aspirin and paracetamol. Most of the study participants thought they were a useful treatment for colds and the flu, and many said they stopped taking them before finishing the course.

In 2015, the Fijian Ministry of Health and Medical Services interviewed five thousand people attending the Hibiscus Festival to get information about Fijians' understanding of antibiotics. It found that many people thought they were used to treat colds and flu, but also headaches, asthma, pregnancy and pain.

What these and other studies show is that people from countries where it's easier to get antibiotics without a prescription are more likely to have misconceptions about what they are useful for.

Each November the WHO runs a campaign called World Antibiotic Awareness Week. Many countries run their own annual campaigns too, usually in winter to discourage people with the symptoms of a mild viral infection not to ask their doctor for antibiotics. Pharmac began running a similar campaign in New Zealand in 1999. But as our rates of rheumatic fever have risen, the message not to see the doctor if you have a sore throat is not the right one. This must be why Pharmac's annual 'Wise use of antibiotics' campaign has disappeared. What's disappointing is that it hasn't been replaced with a more general campaign telling everyone exactly what antibiotics are.

ANTIBIOTIC USE IN MĀORI COMMUNITIES

A surprising finding from the data, is that antibiotic use is low among Māori. This is distinctly at odds with their high burden of infectious diseases. Could it reflect differences for people of different ethnicities in accessing healthcare? Some surveys have shown that this might be the case. One difference is driven by cost. The 2011–12 New Zealand Health Survey found that Māori were more likely than non-Māori not to visit a GP or fill their prescription because of the cost involved.[7] In 2015, GP visits and prescriptions became free for eligible children under thirteen, so hopefully this will remove at least one barrier for children accessing healthcare.

But there are other hidden costs. In the 2011–12 survey, over 100 thousand people said lack of transport prevented them from visiting a GP when they needed to. Others may find it difficult to organise time off work, or make alternative childcare arrangements.

Another barrier is likely to be discrimination and racism. Studies have shown that Māori are less likely to be referred for surgical care and specialist services, and receive lower than expected levels of quality hospital care than non-Māori do.[8] Having a bad experience with healthcare professionals may leave people feeling angry and disempowered and reluctant to seek medical care unless absolutely necessary. And who could blame them?

Dr Lance O'Sullivan is a Kaitaia-based GP whose vision is to democratise healthcare in New Zealand by using technology to deliver high-quality basic health services to communities that need it. The best part of this idea is that the communities manage the technology themselves. O'Sullivan – named New Zealander of the Year in 2014 – has developed the iMOKO programme currently being trialled in Northland. Smart tablets with iMOKO software are placed in early childhood centres, kōhanga reo and primary, intermediate and secondary schools, and approved volunteers are trained to assess children for common health problems. These include sore throats and skin, soft tissue, and dental infections.

The volunteers upload photos and notes about the condition they are presented with, and a cloud-based team uses machine learning to make a prompt and accurate diagnosis and recommend treatment. This is approved by O'Sullivan and his team of doctors wherever they may be at the time. Any necessary prescription and advice on managing the condition is sent back to parents and caregivers using the iMOKO Parent app.

In the short time it has been up and running, iMOKO has successfully delivered healthcare to thousands of Northland children and completely changed their perceptions of what healthcare is and who delivers it. O'Sullivan tells the story of being stopped by an excited young boy as he was about to get into his car. The boy recognised the iMOKO logo on the car door and wanted to tell O'Sullivan about when he had been sick but got better because of the iMOKO iPad. He had no idea that he was talking to the doctor who probably approved his treatment package. And that's just the way O'Sullivan thinks it should be!

7. THE THREATS TO NEW ZEALAND FROM ANTIBIOTIC RESISTANCE

In its first report on antimicrobial resistance around the world, in 2014, the WHO found that resistance is everywhere, and at dangerous levels. It also found that many countries lack any form of surveillance, so it's hard to know how bad the situation is. The report concluded that far from being an apocalyptic fantasy, the post-antibiotic era is a very real possibility for the twenty-first century.

I've recently become friends with an incredible nine-year-old. She was born with only half a diaphragm, and her stomach and bowels don't work. In her short life, she's spent more time in hospital than out of it. She's had many operations, numerous bouts of pneumonia, and several strokes. After all they'd been through, her family didn't think it could get any worse. It did: while she was battling a burst gall bladder and showing no signs of improvement, an antibiotic-resistant superbug called MRSA was found to be rampaging in her bloodstream and growing in the line used to deliver food directly into her body.

She was put in isolation and given antibiotics, and another hole was made in her stomach to replace the line delivering the nutrients she needed. But a little while later the superbug returned, only now resistant to another antibiotic. I'll explain what MRSA is shortly, but first, how does such a superbug develop?

Probably the best way to picture antibiotic resistance is as waves in the ocean. From the very earliest days of antibiotic discovery, every time a new type of antibiotic was taken up, resistant microorganisms emerged and spread like a wave. But there was always another antibiotic on the shelf, so we'd start using that one, and the cycle would repeat itself. The waves of resistance have now become a tsunami, and for some resistant microorganisms, we've no treatments left on the shelf.

Helen Heffernan runs the Antibiotic Reference Laboratory at the Crown institute Environmental Science and Research (ESR). In 2014, she and Deborah Williamson published a paper highlighting the antibiotic-resistant bacteria they believe pose the greatest threat to Kiwi health.[1] We've met one of the bacteria before in this book, but the others might surprise you.

STAPHYLOCOCCUS AUREUS: A SUPERBUG OF OUR OWN MAKING

S. aureus is the versatile bacterium we met earlier that causes all sorts of diseases, from skin and soft tissue infections to food poisoning, pneumonia, meningitis, and blood poisoning (bacteraemia). This is the bacterium for which our rates of disease are among the highest in the developed world, and rising. It's also the bacterium that many healthy people carry around up their noses, on their skin and in their intestines.

S. aureus infections were among the first to be treated with penicillin (a beta-lactam antibiotic) in the 1940s. But even before the drug became widely available, its discoverer, Sir Alexander Fleming, knew that bacteria could develop resistance to it and warned of the dangers of not treating patients for long enough or with doses too low to be fully effective. By the 1950s, penicillin-resistant *S. aureus* was causing outbreaks of disease in hospitals around the world.[2] In 1959, the British pharmaceutical company Beecham developed a new beta-lactam antibiotic called methicillin, also known as meticillin.[3] It became widely used in the 1960s, but strains of methicillin-resistant *S. aureus* were reported as early as 1961. These became known as MRSA. Other beta-lactam antibiotics soon replaced methicillin, but strains of MRSA resist them all.

ESR estimates that about one in ten of the *S. aureus* strains causing infection in New Zealand are MRSA. Annual ESR surveys show that our rates of MRSA infection more than doubled between 2006 and 2011.[4] Those most at risk were aged under five or over sixty-five. Children and young people with MRSA were more likely to be Māori or Pasifika, to live in a deprived neighbourhood, and to catch the infection while going about their day-to-day activities. In contrast, older people were more likely to be Pākehā and to have caught it while in a hospital or some other care facility. What this means is that strains of MRSA are probably circulating in long-term residential care facilities, the residents of which are more likely to be Pākehā.

In 2015, over a thousand people were infected with MRSA. Most of them had skin and soft tissue infections. Almost eight hundred were 'community' patients, that is, individuals who picked up their infection either at home or while going about their day-to-day activities. In New Zealand, doctors will prescribe most patients with a staphylococcal skin infection a cream containing the antibiotic fusidic acid. You might know the cream as Foban. As our rates of skin infections have risen, so have prescriptions for fusidic acid: they quadrupled between 1999 and 2012.[5] And as the number of prescriptions has increased, so has resistance.

The worrying thing is although the antibiotics

are unrelated, resistance to fusidic acid is genetically linked to methicillin resistance, so by using Foban we are actually facilitating the spread of MRSA, infections from which are becoming increasingly difficult to treat.

I started telling you earlier about my little friend with MRSA. When it returned, the doctors removed her infected line, found another place to put a clean one, and treated her with yet another antibiotic. On and on it went until, with just one antibiotic left, the family made the tough choice to remove her line altogether and find another way to feed her. Her weight has plummeted, but she's infection-free for the moment. This is the reality of antibiotic resistance for some vulnerable people in New Zealand right now.

BEWARE THE ENTEROBACTERIACEAE

Klebsiella pneumoniae is a member of a family of bacteria called the Enterobacteriaceae. Another member is *E. coli*. These bacteria are worrying because they are superb at sharing resistance genes with other bacteria, and they can be picked up and carried by people without causing any illness.

As I write this in early 2017, news[6] has just broken that a woman in the US has died after being infected with a strain of *K. pneumoniae* resistant to twenty-six different antibiotics.[7] She spent almost a month in hospital, isolated to stop the bacteria spreading to other patients. The woman had returned home after being in and out of hospital in India; she was in her seventies and had fallen and fractured her leg. She might have responded to one antibiotic, fosfomycin, but it's only approved in the US in tablet form to treat cystitis. She would have needed an intravenous version of the drug.

There was almost a similar story in New Zealand in 2013. 'Teacher NZ's first victim of superbug' screamed the headline.[8] 'He died fighting a superbug that no antibiotic in the world could touch,' the article went on. In fact, sixty-eight-year-old Brian Pool died from the complications of a brain haemorrhage, suffered while living in Vietnam. But he did test positive in Wellington for antibiotic-resistant *K. pneumoniae*.

It didn't kill him. It was just living inside him. But if it had got into the bloodstreams or lungs of other vulnerable patients, doctors wouldn't have had any antibiotics to treat them with. That's why Pool spent the last six months of his life quarantined in hospital, unable to be hugged by his family or to sit out in the courtyard and feel the sunshine on his face. A personal tragedy, and massively expensive for our healthcare system.

Many Enterobacteriaceae were initially sensitive to penicillin but soon became resistant by producing an enzyme called a beta-lactamase that destroys the antibiotic. In the 1960s, the

American pharmaceutical company Eli Lilly and Co introduced a class of antibiotics called cephalosporins that are impervious to beta-lactamase enzymes. This favoured bacteria that could produce enzymes (called extended-spectrum beta-lactamases, or ESBLs) able to destroy these antibiotics too. Each year, ESBL-producing strains of *E. coli* and *K. pneumoniae* are isolated from thousands of New Zealanders of all ages.[9] About half of these people are just carrying the bacteria without any problems. But the rest can end up with pneumonia, blood poisoning or a urinary tract infection.

The good news is that they can be treated with another class of antibiotics called carbapenems. The bad news is that these medicines usually need to be given intravenously in hospital. In other words, they are inconvenient and expensive.

I'm sure you won't be surprised to hear that the use of carbapenems has supported the emergence of Enterobacteriaceae that produce yet more antibiotic-destroying enzymes, called carbapenemases. While still rare in New Zealand (we had just thirty-eight cases in 2016),[10] carbapenem-resistant bacteria are widespread India – probably because of the easy access people have to antibiotics there, as well as the problems I mentioned with environmental contamination from their manufacture.

It's not just India, though. Carbapenem-resistant bacteria are on the rise worldwide. This is why it's standard practice for hospitals in New Zealand to swab people if they've been hospitalised overseas. If they are found to be carrying these resistant bacteria, they'll be placed in isolation. Most of the thirty-eight cases we had in 2016 were people who had been hospitalised in, or had travelled to, India. Others had been in hospital in Turkey, Dubai, China and the Philippines. In 2015, a New Zealand tourist transferred to Christchurch Hospital was found to be carrying seven different carbapenem-resistant bacteria![11] That person had spent two months in hospital in Romania.

If you're breathing a sigh of relief because the countries I've just mentioned aren't on your list of holiday destinations, American researchers have just reported that carbapenem-resistant Enterobacteriaceae isolated from patients in Massachusetts and California might be spreading among healthy people out in the community.[12] These superbugs are probably more widespread than we think.

Nowadays when a doctor has a patient with a carbapenemase-producing strain of *E. coli* or *K. pneumoniae* they have to fall back on antibiotics discovered decades ago but rarely used because of their toxicity. Colistin is one of these 'last resort' antibiotics. But guess what? It's starting to fail too. While some bacteria can mutate to become colistin-resistant during treatment, in late 2015 researchers in China discovered a form of colistin resistance that can spread between different species of bacteria.[13] It turns out that while doctors had abandoned colistin, the agricultural industry had not, and China is one of the biggest users.

The researchers isolated colistin-resistant *E. coli* from more than a quarter of the samples of chicken and pork meat they tested from Chinese supermarkets. And it's not just China. Colistin-resistant bacteria have been isolated from chicken meat for sale in Europe too.[14] Now these strains are turning up in people. This is another stark example of why we need a 'One Health' approach to tackling infectious diseases and antibiotic resistance.

GONORRHOEA – ANOTHER HIDDEN DANGER

There was a case in the UK recently where a man went to a sexual health clinic after experiencing two weeks of a burning sensation when he peed and fluid leaking from the tip of his penis.[15] The clinic found the bacterium *Neisseria gonorrhoeae* living in the urethra and throat of this man, who'd not long returned from Japan. He had gonorrhoea, also known as the clap.

The routine treatment used to be tablets of ciprofloxacin. But as more and more strains have become resistant to this antibiotic, treatment has had to change to something less convenient and more expensive: an injection of ceftriaxone and a dose of azithromycin tablets. The man was given his antibiotics and instructed to return two weeks later. Fresh swabs showed he still had bacteria in his throat. But after getting his results, the man didn't come back for more treatment for another three months!

When he did finally return, he was given higher doses of ceftriaxone and azithromycin. This time the treatment worked. But how many people might he have given gonorrhoea to in the meantime?

Like chlamydia, gonorrhoea can be transmitted during vaginal, anal and oral sex, and from an infected mother to her baby during childbirth. While most men will have symptoms when they are infected, half of infected women may have none at all. Just like chlamydia, if left untreated, gonorrhoea can cause inflammation in the testes in men, pelvic inflammatory disease in women, and all of the associated complications I mentioned earlier, including infertility. It can also spread to joints and heart valves.

Gonorrhoea is another disease that isn't notifiable in New Zealand, so doctors don't have to report cases they see. The best estimates put our rate at seventy cases per 100 thousand people in 2014, three-quarters of them in the 15–29 age group. While we're not quite topping the charts this time, our rates are rising. And gonorrhoea is also becoming resistant to antibiotic treatment. Ceftriaxone-resistant strains of *N. gonorrhoeae* have been reported in Australia, the UK, France, Spain and Japan. Azithromycin-resistant strains are even more widespread.

When ESR looked at antibiotic resistance in *N. gonorrhoeae* strains from infected Kiwis in 2015 it found that about 10 per cent were either resistant or on their way to being resistant to azithromycin.[16] A very small number of strains were also on their way to being ceftriaxone-resistant too. Once these antibiotics stop working, the options for treatment are very limited.

One concern is that most labs in New Zealand test for *N. gonorrhoeae* by looking for the presence of the bacteria's genetic material, rather than culturing the microbes on a Petri dish. The genetic tests are much faster, so this makes sense. But the problem with the standard tests is that they don't tell us anything about what antibiotics the bacteria are resistant to. For that, we need to grow the bacteria too. This means that ESR can't even do its antibiotic-resistance tests on all the strains of *N. gonorrhoeae* causing infection.

The case of the young British man shows just how easily people can spread these infectious microbes around. From Japan to the UK, in one easy flight. We Kiwis love to travel, and fewer than half of our sexually active young people say they use condoms.[17] That's a frightening combination when it comes to antibiotic-resistant gonorrhoea.

THE DISEASE THAT NEVER REALLY WENT AWAY

If we want an example of the dangers of ignoring public health crises just because they are happening elsewhere, tuberculosis is it. More commonly known as TB, this disease has been with us for thousands of years, even identified in mummies from Egypt and Peru. Until the 1880s, most people thought it was a hereditary disease that tended to strike people in their twenties and thirties. Known as consumption then, it was often romanticised in literature. No horrible, rapid death accompanied by vomiting and diarrhoea – instead, consumptives were portrayed as thin and pale, discreetly coughing blood into their handkerchiefs, with time enough to draw up their wills and make peace with friends and family. In her 1847 novel *Wuthering Heights*, Emily Brontë describes her consumptive heroine as 'rather thin, but young, and fresh-complexioned, and her eyes sparkled as bright as diamonds'.

That the very slow-growing *Mycobacterium tuberculosis* was destroying the consumptive's lungs wasn't clear until 1882. That was the year that Dr Robert Koch (1843–1910) reported he had isolated the bacterium. Now we know that TB is spread mainly through the air, when infectious people cough, sneeze or even sing. We also think that people can become infected by breathing in as few as ten bacteria.

Most of those infected won't show any symptoms and aren't infectious. The bacteria will be hiding in their lungs, waiting. We call this latent TB. It's estimated that 1.7 billion people around the world have it.[18] That's roughly a quarter of everyone alive today. People with latent TB have about a one-in-ten chance of progressing to active disease. This likelihood increases as they age, become malnourished, or become immunocompromised. Active TB is infectious, and fatal if untreated.

Before the discovery of antibiotics, those who could afford it spent time in sanatoria in the hope that fresh air and sunlight would cure them. Some sanatoria also offered forms of treatment such as collapsing parts of a patient's lungs. It's not clear whether people were ever actually cured at such places, but at least infectious patients were removed from their communities.

The first effective anti-TB antibiotic, streptomycin, was discovered in the mid-1940s. Researchers soon realised, however, that it didn't kill *M. tuberculosis*, just stopped it from growing, and that the bacterium could mutate to become resistant. It wasn't until the 1950s and 60s that antibiotics capable of actually killing

M. tuberculosis were discovered: isoniazid, pyrazinamide, cycloserine, ethambutol and rifampicin (also known as rifampin).

The standard treatment for TB became a gruelling cocktail of antibiotics and remains so to this day. An intensive eight-week phase (daily doses of isoniazid, rifampicin, pyrazinamide and ethambutol) is followed by daily or thrice-weekly doses of isoniazid and rifampicin for another eighteen weeks. A few years ago, I hosted a visit from a man in his nineties who was interested in seeing our new TB research lab. He told me about being treated for TB as a younger man, all the pills he'd had to take, and the side-effects that made him very ill. He was aghast when I told him we still relied on those same medicines to treat TB today.

As awful as those medicines are, they helped to bring TB under control in Europe and the US, where it had been one of the leading causes of death in the nineteenth century. By the mid-twentieth century it was becoming increasingly rare in high-income countries. But other parts of the world were less fortunate, and *M. tuberculosis* continued to thrive and spread in conditions of extreme poverty – so much so, that it is still one of the top ten causes of death worldwide, killing 1.8 million people in 2015. That's more than die from HIV and malaria. It's estimated that there were more than 10 million new cases contracted around the world in 2015.

Wherever patients haven't had access to the right cocktail of drugs for the right amount of time or didn't finish their treatment because of the side-effects, antibiotic resistance has emerged. In the 1990s, strains of *M. tuberculosis* resistant to rifampicin and isoniazid (referred to as 'multi-drug resistant', or MDR for short) were found everywhere people looked for them, even causing outbreaks in American hospitals and prisons. It's estimated that almost half a million people developed MDR-TB in 2015, with 190 thousand dying as a result. India, China and Russia accounted for about half these cases.

We've had a very small number of MDR-TB cases in New Zealand too – fifteen between 2010 and 2014. MDR-TB takes even longer to treat than regular TB, using a bigger cocktail of less effective 'second-line' drugs, some of which have to be given intravenously. In countries that can afford it, patients are kept in isolation in hospital.

According to the WHO, only one in five people with MDR-TB are getting the right treatment. It's no surprise then that strains of *M. tuberculosis* have become resistant to those second-line drugs too. We call these strains 'extensively drug-resistant', or XDR for short. As for the strains that have become resistant to all first-line and second-line anti-TB drugs, we call them totally drug-resistant (TDR).

Some new anti-TB drugs are being developed.

New Zealand has played a part in this research effort through the work of Distinguished Professor Bill Denny and his colleagues at Auckland University.[19] But the WHO estimates that to fully bring the TB epidemic under control in low- and middle-income countries will cost more than $US8 billion a year, and in 2016 they were almost $US2 billion short. The WHO says that at least an extra $US1 billion a year is needed for research.

Most of the six hundred people diagnosed with TB in New Zealand each year (about three hundred with latent disease, three hundred active) were born overseas, or live with someone who was. Most, but not all. In 2010, the country had its first case of XDR-TB when a young man in Dunedin went to see his GP because fluid was leaking out of an enlarged lymph node on his neck.[20] That fluid turned out to be XDR *M. tuberculosis*.

The man was hospitalised and treated with a daily combination of seven different medicines. The hospital pharmacy even had to import some of the drugs from the US after supplies in New Zealand ran out. Over a month later he was sent home on another cocktail of drugs, which he had to take for eighteen months. The medicines alone cost $10,000 a month. Unlike many cases of XDR-TB, this one had a happy ending – the man fully recovered and, luckily for the people of Dunedin, his type of XDR-TB wasn't airborne.

M. tuberculosis is one of the bacteria we study in my lab, and a few years ago, I gave a presentation about our research to a group of wealthy retired women in Auckland. I talked a little about the six hundred people diagnosed with TB in 2013. Afterwards, one of the women came up and quietly told me that she had been one of them. I'll never forget what she said next: 'I was horrified when my doctor told me I had TB. I said he must have made a mistake. Women like me don't get TB!'

No matter how wealthy you are, if you are breathing and come into contact with someone who is infectious, you can get TB.

8. TIME FOR ACTION

Having read this far, I hope that you will have been convinced that infectious diseases are a problem not just globally, but also right here in New Zealand. I also hope that, like Margaret Chan and Lord O'Neill, you will see that unless we act now, antimicrobial resistance threatens to undo many of the medical achievements of the last century. Now the question should be, what can we do about all this? And, perhaps more important, what can *you* do about it?

One place we can start is by tackling the infectious microbes that are already a burden to our society and healthcare system: *Campylobacter* and other food- and water-borne microorganisms, *Staphylococcus aureus*, *Streptococcus pyogenes*, *Chlamydia trachomatis* and *Mycobacterium tuberculosis*. These are very different microbes, spread in different ways, so there is no simple one-size-fits-all solution. But that's no excuse for inaction. The stakes are too high.

There are lots of ways that you can personally contribute to protecting yourself and others from infectious diseases. You can learn to wash and dry your hands properly.[1] You can steer clear of drinking unpasteurised (so-called 'raw') milk and eating unwashed fruit and vegetables. You can keep your raw meat away from your fresh vegetables. You can make sure you properly cook any meat you prepare. You can avoid swimming in our rivers and lakes. You can get vaccinated. If you are sexually active, you can use condoms and dental dams.

Whatever your age, you can go and get tested to make sure you aren't asymptomatically carrying a sexually transmitted infection. Because it's not just teenagers that get chlamydia or gonorrhoea. Most important of all, if you ever catch yourself thinking that you aren't the kind of person who's likely to get MRSA/TB/gonorrhoea/etc., stop and remind yourself that you are wrong. They are called infectious diseases for a reason.

Tackling the rising rates is more complicated and requires us to start asking some hard questions about what we value as a society. If it's that we should be able to swim in our rivers and lakes without getting sick, then we need to think seriously about curbing the impact of the agricultural industry on our health and environment. If we value the idea that every child should be able to reach their full potential, then we need to think seriously about the impact that rising income inequality and a severe lack of affordable, warm, dry housing is having on our nation's health. According to the Office of the Children's Commissioner, 14 per cent of children experienced income poverty in 1982.[2] The most recent data, from 2015, has that figure at 28 per cent. Let that sink in for a moment. Almost a third of Kiwi kids are growing up in poverty.

In 1993, New Zealand ratified the United Nations Convention on the Rights of the Child, which states that all children are of equal worth and should have equal opportunities.[3] Our government also agreed that laws and actions affecting children should put their interests first and benefit them in the best possible way. Let's see whether that has been happening.

In December 2012, the Children's Commissioner's Expert Advisory Group on Solutions to Child Poverty recommended the introduction of a housing 'warrant of fitness' to ensure that rental houses are well ventilated, insulated and heated.[4] In 2016, the government responded by passing the Residential Tenancies Amendment Bill. This law requires rental homes to have smoke detectors fitted and to be insulated to the standards set in 1978.[5] Not the current standards, but inferior standards almost four decades old. Standards for heating and ventilation were also missing.

In this regard, I think it's safe to say that the government hasn't put our children's interests first. Instead, the most vulnerable are going to continue living in cold, damp, mouldy houses. They will keep being admitted to our hospitals with infectious diseases. In essence, we are reaping what New Zealand's neoliberal economic policies of the 1990s sowed. And current policies don't seem to be changing anything.

TACKLING ANTIBIOTIC-RESISTANT 'SUPERBUGS'

In the previous chapter, I described the major threats we face from antibiotic-resistant microbes: homegrown MRSA, and the importation of almost untreatable strains of *M. tuberculosis*, *N. gonorrhoea*, *K. pneumonia* and *E. coli*. What can we do about this crisis? Closing our borders isn't a solution. Not unless all New Zealanders are willing to stop travelling too. And we travel a lot. According to Statistics New Zealand, in 2014 there were more than 700 thousand overseas departures from Auckland airport by resident New Zealanders going on holiday.[6] Another 600 thousand were going to visit friends and relatives abroad. Each of those trips is an opportunity to bring back an invisible infectious passenger.

To tackle the crisis, we need to better manage the antibiotics we have by using them more wisely and sparingly. We also need to discover new classes of antibiotics and new ways to diagnose and treat infectious diseases.

In 2015, the WHO published its 'global action plan' for tackling antimicrobial resistance.[7] Objectives include improving awareness and understanding of antimicrobial resistance, optimising the use of antimicrobial agents in people and animals, and increasing investment in new medicines, diagnostic tools, vaccines, and other interventions. New Zealand has made a commitment to the WHO to have a national strategic antimicrobial resistance action plan in place by May 2017,[8] and a cross-agency group has been brought together to develop this. We'll have to wait and see how many of the WHO's objectives New Zealand's plan addresses, and how the government responds.

FUNDING FOR INFECTIOUS DISEASES RESEARCH

Throughout the country, researchers are working to understand how infectious microbes tick, and to find chinks in their armour. Others of us are trying to discover and develop new antimicrobial compounds and therapies. I'll come back to this later. The biggest barrier we face in making progress is money. Or rather, a lack of it.

I'll never forget a chat I had with my brother a few years ago, about how scientific research is funded in universities. A crowdfunding initiative called the SciFund Challenge had been launched, and I set out to raise $4,000 towards one of the projects in my lab.[9] In the space of a month I raised $6,000 from seventy-nine friends and strangers around the world. This was a drop in the bucket (the project cost hundreds of thousands of dollars), but I was curious to see how I'd go.

When my brother asked me why I would bother raising small amounts of money online when I was paid by my university to do research, I realised for the first time that most people don't know how research is funded. Why should they? Let me explain how it usually works. University academics are paid to teach and do research, but most universities don't just hand out money to pay for the actual research itself. That's okay if it involves the academic thinking and writing, but if the academic needs people to do experiments, or has to buy things like Petri dishes and chemicals, or needs to pay to access expensive bits of equipment either here or overseas, then they have to raise the money themselves.

A recent study of medical researchers in Australia found that it took them thirty-eight working days on average to prepare an application to the National Health and Medical Research Council.[10]

For just one funding round, that was the equivalent of 550 working years of researchers' time, costing $A66 million in salary. The year of the study, only 21 per cent of proposals were successful, meaning that 434.5 working years, and more than $A52 million, was lost by the research community.

Just to be clear, the time and money weren't lost because the researchers were writing bad applications. They were lost because there was only enough money in the pot to fund 21 per cent of the proposals, and a judging panel had to choose between them. Research has recently shown that judging panels are unable to differentiate between good applications.[11]

Here in New Zealand, there are several different places medical researchers like me can apply for funding to pay for our experiments. One of these is charities that support medical research, the biggest funders of which are the Cancer Society (about $3 million a year), the Auckland Medical Research Foundation ($2.6 million) and Cure Kids ($2.4 million). Next are the Neurological Foundation (about $1.3 million a year), the Genesis Oncology Trust ($1 million) and the Heart Foundation ($800,000). Smaller amounts are administered by the Otago Medical Research Foundation ($300,000) and the Maurice and Phyllis Paykel Trust ($250,000). Of the $12 million these charities gave to medical research in 2016, just 3 per cent went on projects involving infectious diseases. That's less than half a million dollars.

Why is there is so little philanthropic support for infectious diseases research? One of the main reasons is that no charities are dedicated to this area of health. How many friends do you know who have done a charity walk or run to support cancer research? I imagine it's more than those who did one for MRSA! But even if we look at charities that fund all medical areas, like the Auckland Medical Research Foundation, just 5 to 10 per cent has been awarded to infectious diseases research. All of these charities get many more applications each year than they can fund, so they have to make tough decisions about what to support.

The government is by far the biggest funder of medical research through a variety of schemes but New Zealand spends less than the OECD average on research and development,[12] so competition for funding is fierce, with success rates for many schemes below 10 per cent. About half the money awarded to researchers – sometimes even more – goes straight to their institution to help cover overheads and salary.

The bulk of funding comes from the Health Research Council, which between 2012 and 2016 allocated $365 million for 'applied' medical research that will improve human health within a few years. Less than 10 per cent was awarded to infectious diseases research. Thirty million dollars might sound like a lot, but it doesn't go very far, funding fewer than twenty projects over five years.

Then there's the Marsden Fund. Over the past five years, medical researchers have submitted more than five hundred applications. Forty-six were funded, seven of which were related to infectious diseases.

The government's Endeavour Fund allocates roughly $180 million a year to commercially applicable research. Only a very small part of that will be spent on medical research, as the fund covers all research fields and is mainly intended for projects that will grow our economy. Saying that, 5 per cent is set aside for projects that can help 'deliver better public services and improve the quality of life and wellbeing for New Zealanders'.[13]

The government also distributes some of the Lotteries Commission's profits to medical research via the Lottery Grants Board. Between 2011 and 2014, over $11 million was allocated; less than 8 per cent went to infectious diseases.

Another way that the government funds research is through the Centres of Research Excellence, a scheme that began in 2002. These virtual centres bring together people from all over the country to build a critical mass of expertise in particular areas. The Tertiary Education Commission funds them to train the scientific workforce through PhD scholarships. The centres are decided through a competitive bid process every six years. There are currently three health-related centres, including one dedicated to brain research and another to developing innovative medical devices and technologies.

In 2006, Professor Kurt Krause of Otago University led a bid to create a Centre for Molecular Biodefence against Infectious Pathogens that would develop 'diagnostics, antimicrobials, and vaccines to address important problems caused by infectious diseases in New Zealand'.[14] Its research would include bacterial resistance and evolution, antimicrobials, antifungals, and the genetics of disease susceptibility.

Krause had pulled together sixty-five researchers from four universities and three Crown research institutes for the bid. We'll never know why the proposal failed. Perhaps there just wasn't enough money in the pot. Or maybe those reviewing it didn't believe infectious diseases were a big enough problem, and the fact that they were already included as a research area in one of the three current health-related centres – the Maurice Wilkins Centre for Molecular Biodiscovery[15] – was sufficient. Wilkins Centre researchers are also studying cancer, diabetes and metabolic diseases, and new technology platforms.

It takes about a decade to bring new drugs from

the lab to the clinic. I can't help but wonder what we've lost by not funding Krause's centre more than ten years ago. Even back then, the first theme proposed was antibiotic resistance. A similar bid in 2014 also failed.

NATIONAL SCIENCE CHALLENGES

The UK has been extremely proactive in addressing the issue of antimicrobial resistance, developing a five-year strategic plan in 2013.[16] In 2014, a charity called Antibiotic Research UK was launched with the aim of raising enough money to bring at least one new antibiotic to market by the early 2020s.[17] It needs to raise £550,000 in 2017 to fund its mission. Also in 2014, it was announced that the UK public had chosen to prevent the rise of antibiotic resistance as the focus of a very special prize.[18]

Seeking to dominate the world's oceans, the British government in 1714 offered, by act of parliament, an enormous financial reward for solving the greatest scientific challenge of that time: how to pinpoint a ship's location at sea by knowing its longitude. To commemorate the three hundredth anniversary of the Longitude Act, in 2013 the government reinstated the Longitude Committee, which spent a year consulting with the UK public and scientific community to devise a short list of the scientific challenges of our time. They came up with six, from flying without damaging the environment, to ensuring that everyone has nutritious, sustainable food and access to safe and clean water.

The public were then asked to choose from the six the one they thought should be the subject of a modern-day Longitude Prize – and they chose tackling antibiotic resistance. The winner of the £10 million prize will be the person or group who, before 2019, develops a diagnostic test that can rapidly identify if a patient doesn't need antibiotics, or, if they do, which one should be used.

In this country, the government in 2012 announced a $60 million initiative called the National Science Challenges,[19] along with a TV and web campaign called the Great New Zealand Science Project.[20] Launching the initiatives, the Minister for Science and Innovation, Steven Joyce, said:

We are keen for the public and the science community to tell us what they think New Zealand's most important science challenges are over the next five to ten years, so we can focus our investment on solving these challenges for the benefit of New Zealand. [21]

The Great New Zealand Science Project featured short videos of eight scientists explaining their research as examples of the kinds of things the challenges could focus on, and the public were asked to vote for the video they believed was in the most important area. I was one of the scientists featured, and the video of me talking about infectious diseases got the most votes.[22] Seems like beating the superbugs struck a chord with the public!

In early 2013, Joyce announced that an elevenperson 'Peak Panel' appointed and chaired by the Prime Minister's Chief Science Adviser, Sir Peter Gluckman,[23] had been tasked with recommending between six and ten final challenges for the government to approve.[24] Later that year, ten were announced; an eleventh was added in 2014.

What's been funded is important, as the government has indicated that other funders, like the Health Research Council, will be moving to align their research investments to support the challenges. This means that almost $1.6 billion of funding will be invested in the National Science Challenges.

Four of the challenges are health-related,[25] and at first glance it looks as though infectious diseases research fits into the remit of the ones focused on 'A better start' and 'Healthier lives'. However, the panel specifically excluded infectious diseases from those challenges, and the 'Ageing well' challenge too. They are to focus only on non-communicable diseases.

The panel was tasked with choosing the challenges on the criteria of additionality (that is, what would they add to the health science sector) and current scientific capacity and capability. The idea that a challenge focused on infectious diseases doesn't meet the criteria of additionality sounds crazy to me. In a country with rising rates of infectious diseases, and a worldwide antibiotic-resistance crisis that threatens us all, I can't think of a better topic for a National Science Challenge. In fact, such a challenge would have plugged a massive gap in resourcing.

At the press conference announcing the challenges, I asked Gluckman why infectious diseases had been excluded. He replied that the challenges focused on the areas in which New Zealand had capacity and capability. In other words, to the Peak Panel our country doesn't have a critical mass of people working in infectious diseases research.

It's not hard to see how the panel reached this conclusion. First, there was no infectious diseases expert among its members. Instead there were several experts in non-communicable diseases. Looking at the summary of submissions from the science community that the panel reviewed, it seems as though researchers studying infectious diseases didn't engage with the process.[26] With no voice at the table, and no submissions from the esteemed professors actively working in the area, infectious diseases were left out in the cold.

For a couple of years after the Great New Zealand Science Project campaign appeared on TV, people would stop me on the street asking if I'd won the money for my research. I think they'd be surprised to hear that the science I do is excluded.

DOWN BUT NOT OUT

By now you are probably wondering if New Zealand has any researchers fighting the superbugs! Rest assured we do. After almost a decade working on various infectious microbes at Imperial College London, in 2009 I moved to New Zealand with my Kiwi husband and daughter. My speciality area is making bacteria glow in the dark – like glow worms! The bacteria will only glow when they are alive, and measuring light is quicker and easier than waiting for living bacteria to grow on Petri dishes. Throughout my career, my lab and I have made glowing versions of many of the bacteria mentioned in this book, including *E. coli*, *S. aureus*, *S. pyogenes*, and *M. tuberculosis*.

Until about three years ago, my research had focused on using these glowing bacteria and laboratory mice to understand more about the interactions between bacteria and their hosts. A chance meeting with fungi expert Dr Peter Buchanan (at a Lego exhibition of all places!) changed that. He told me about a collection of about 10 thousand fungi kept at Landcare Research, another of New Zealand's Crown research institutes. As far as Buchanan was aware, the fungi in the collection had never been tested to see if they made antibiotics. New Zealand is famous for its flightless birds – do we also have fungi producing antibiotics able to kill the almost untreatable superbugs?

My lab is now working with chemist Associate Professor Brent Copp and Buchanan's colleague Dr Bevan Weir to find new antibiotics from those 10 thousand fungi. So far, we've looked at about three hundred and found some able to kill MRSA and *M. tuberculosis*. Fingers crossed that they turn out to be making new antibiotics. And if they aren't, we still have more than 9,500 left to test!

Of course, I'm not the only scientist in the country researching infectious microbes. Describing all of them would take another book, but here are just a few others who are right now trying to discover new antibiotics, and new ways to treat infectious diseases.

At Massey University, Dr Heather Hendrickson is the first international collaborator on an American project – supported by the Howard Hughes Medical Institute's Science Education Alliance – looking for new bacteriophages, viruses that infect only specific strains of bacteria. Currently used overseas to prevent meat contamination, they have massive potential as an alternative to antibiotics. Unlike antibiotics, because they are so specific, they don't affect all the helpful bacteria living inside us. Hendrickson and her students are searching soil and water samples to find new bacteriophages capable of killing medically and agriculturally important bacteria.

Massey University is also home to the Infectious Diseases Research Centre, a group of researchers headed by Professor Nigel French with a focus on 'One Health' and food- and water-borne diseases.

At Otago University, Kurt Krause heads the Webster Centre for Infectious Diseases where Dr Joanna Kirman and her team are trying to understand our immune system, in order to develop better TB vaccines; and Professor Greg Cook and his team are looking for new drugs to treat TB.

At Victoria University, Associate Professor David Ackerley, Dr Jeremy Owen and their team are trying to reengineer some antibiotics to see if they can get around the ways bacteria have of resisting them. They also hope to 'fish' out any unknown genes that bacteria use to make antibiotics, directly from New Zealand soils.

At Auckland University, Associate Professor Thomas Proft and his team are seeking to develop new vaccines, while Associate Professor Simon Swift and the Biocide Toolbox team are trying to develop surfaces that microbes can't attach to or grow on. That would be useful for all sorts of things, including preventing infection after surgery.

In reality, many of us working to beat the antibiotic-resistance crisis are struggling to raise the money we need for our research. So, what can you do about this? Some suggestions:

- Write to the Finance Minister and ask for more money to be spent on scientific research.
- Write to the Prime Minister, Finance Minister, Science Minister and Chief Science Advisor and ask for a new National Science Challenge dedicated to antibiotic resistance.
- Donate to Cure Kids, one of the few charities actively funding research in this area.
- Run a marathon, or hold a bake sale, for any number of the researchers working on infectious diseases.
- Give up a coffee a week and make a standing donation to support a research group.
- If you need a gift for someone, buy them a T-shirt or something from our online shop,[27] or sponsor one of our 10 thousand fungi.[28]
- Or you could follow in the UK's footsteps and volunteer to help launch a charity dedicated to discovering new antibiotics.

A future without effective antibiotics and other antimicrobials will affect us all, rich and poor, young and old. Will *you* help? The stakes are enormous, and time is running out.

LIST OF ACRONYMS

AIDS	Acquired Immune Deficiency Syndrome
BRICS	Brazil, Russia, India, China and South Africa
CDDEP	Centre for Disease Dynamics, Economics and Policy
DHB	District Health Board
DNA	deoxyribonucleic acid
EPHA	European Public Health Alliance
ESBL	extended-spectrum beta-lactamase
ESR	Environmental Science and Research
FDA	Food and Drug Administration
HIV	Human Immunodeficiency Virus
IVF	in vitro fertilisation
MPI	Ministry for Primary Industries
MRSA	methicillin-resistant *Staphylococcus aureus*
OECD	Organisation for Economic Co-operation and Development
PBP	penicillin-binding protein
PHARMAC	Pharmaceutical Management Agency

RNA	ribonucleic acid
SCCmec	Staphylococcal chromosome cassette *mec*
SU	standard unit
TB	Tuberculosis
WHO	World Health Organization

APPENDIX: QUIZ ANSWERS FROM PAGE 15

DISEASES

AIDS	Acquired Immune Deficiency Syndrome caused by the Human Immunodeficiency Virus (HIV)
Aspergillosis	Caused by the fungus *Aspergillus fumigatus* and its relatives
Bilharzia	Also known as schistosomiasis. Caused by parasitic worms (flukes) called *Schistosoma*
Botulism	Caused by the bacterium *Clostridium botulinum*
Gonorrhoea	Caused by the bacterium *Neisseria gonorrhoeae*
Impetigo	Caused by the bacteria *Streptococcus pyogenes* (also known as Group A Strep) and *Staphylococcus aureus*
Influenza	Commonly known as the flu. Caused by the Influenza virus

Malaria	Caused by the parasitic protozoa *Plasmodium falciparum* and its relatives
Measles	Caused by the Measles virus
Meningitis	Inflammation of the protective membranes covering the brain and spinal cord. Can be caused by bacteria like *Neisseria meningitidis* and *Streptococcus pneumoniae*, viruses like varicella zoster (chickenpox) and mumps, as well as some fungi and parasites
Pneumonia	Inflammation of the lungs that can be caused by viruses like Influenza and respiratory syncytial virus (RSV), bacteria like *Streptococcus pneumoniae* and *Klebsiella pneumoniae*, as well as some fungi and parasites
Polio	Caused by Poliovirus
Rheumatic fever	Caused by the bacterium *Streptococcus pyogenes*

Ringworm	Caused by fungi of the *Trichophyton*, *Microsporum*, and *Epidermophyton* families
Syphilis	Caused by the bacterium *Treponema pallidum*
Tonsillitis	Caused by the bacterium *Streptococcus pyogenes*
Toxoplasmosis	Caused by the parasite *Toxoplasma gondii*
Tuberculosis (TB)	Caused by the bacterium *Mycobacterium tuberculosis*

MICROORGANISMS

Campylobacter jejuni	Bacterium responsible for campylobacteriosis
Chlamydia trachomatis	Bacterium responsible for chlamydia
Giardia lamblia	Parasite responsible for giardiasis
Haemophilus influenzae	Bacterium that can cause a range of infections
Hepatitis A	Virus that causes hepatitis
HIV	Human Immunodeficiency Virus responsible for AIDS

MRSA	Bacterium (Methicillin-resistant *Staphylococcus aureus*) responsible for a range of infections
Staphylococcus aureus	Bacterium
Zika	Virus responsible for microcephaly, a condition in which babies are born with small heads

NOTES

Chapter 1

1. Bacteria without a second membrane layer around their peptidoglycan are called Gram-positive, while ones that have this membrane are called Gram-negative. The name comes from a test devised by Hans Christian Gram (1853–1938) based on the ability of bacteria to stain with a dye called crystal violet.

2. R. Sender, S. Fuchs and R. Milo, 'Revised Estimates for the Number of Human and Bacteria Cells in the Body', *PLoS Biol*, 14, 8 (2016), e1002533, https://doi.org/10.1371/journal.pbio.1002533

3. If you thought the blue whale was the largest creature on Earth, think again. That title may well belong to the 'humongous fungus', a colony of honey fungus (*Armillaria solidipes*) growing in the Blue Mountains in Oregon, US, whose mycelium is thought to cover an area of over 9.5 square kilometres, and could be several thousand years old (Nic Fleming, 'The Largest Living Thing on Earth is a Humongous Fungus', BBC, 19 November 2014, www.bbc.com/earth/story/20141114-the-biggest-organism-in-the-world [accessed 16 March 2017]).

4. If you are wondering why some of the organisms listed are italicised and others not, it's because we use a system called binomial nomenclature when writing their scientific names. Species are identified by a combination of two words, which take Latin grammatical form even if they are words based on other languages. The first word identifies the genus to which the species belongs, while the second word identifies the species within the genus. The words are always italicised and the first word always starts with a capital letter. The convention is to write out the organism's genus name in full the first time it's used and then to abbreviate it after that. So, *Staphylococcus aureus* becomes *S. aureus*. To complicate matters, the names commonly used to refer to specific viruses tend

not to use their species name but a common name that often relates to the disease they cause or where they were first identified: Hepatitis A, Ebola. That's why they aren't italicised.

Chapter 2

1. Institute for Health Metrics and Evaluation, 'GBD Compare', http://vizhub.healthdata.org/gbd-compare (accessed 16 March 2017).

2. M.G. Baker et al., 'Increasing Incidence of Serious Infectious Diseases and Inequalities in New Zealand: A National Epidemiological Study', *Lancet*, 379, 9821 (2012), pp.1112–19, https://doi.org/10.1016/S0140-6736(11)61780-7.

3. Ministry of Health, 'Publicly Funded Hospital Discharges – 1 July 2013 to 30 June 2014', 28 July 2016, www.health.govt.nz/publication/publicly-funded-hospital-discharges-1-july-2013-30-june-2014 (accessed 16 March 2017).

4. Figure.NZ, 'Deaths Caused by Infectious Diseases in New Zealand: By Agent', Statistics New Zealand, https://figure.nz/chart/h81I77EvWrRQYOaf (accessed 16 March 2017).

5. Figure.NZ, 'Hospitalisations Caused by Infectious Diseases in New Zealand: By Agent', Statistics New Zealand, https://figure.nz/chart/VazjU29wIocilyT8 (accessed 16 March 2017).

6. Figure.NZ, 'Hospitalisations Caused by Infectious Diseases in New Zealand: By Category', Statistics New Zealand, https://figure.nz/chart/5fecH09MPQqjAy6q (accessed 16 March 2017).

7. D.A. Williamson et al., '*Staphylococcus aureus* Infections in New Zealand, 2000–2011', *Emerg Infect Dis*, 20, 7 (2014), pp.1156–61, https://doi.org/10.3201/eid2007.131923.

8. D.A. Williamson et al., 'Clinical and Molecular Epidemiology of Community-Onset Invasive *Staphylococcus aureus* Infection in New Zealand Children', *Epidemiol Infect*, 142, 8 (2014), pp.1713–21, https://doi.org/10.1017/S0950268814000053.

9. C. O'Sullivan and M.G. Baker, 'Skin Infections in Children in a New Zealand Primary Care Setting: Exploring Beneath the Tip of the Iceberg', *NZ Med J*, 125, 1351 (2012), pp.70–79.

10. D.A. Williamson et al., 'Incidence, Trends

and Demographics of *Staphylococcus aureus* Infections in Auckland, New Zealand, 2001–2011', *BMC Infect Dis*, 13 (2013), p.569.

11 Michelle Robinson, 'Family Counts Blessings After Superbug Scare', *Dominion Post*, 19 May 2013, www.stuff.co.nz/dominion-post/news/8690893/Family-counts-blessings-after-superbug-scare (accessed 16 March 2017).

12 Joanne Black, 'The Rise of Necrotising Fasciitis', *The Listener*, 17 December 2011, www.noted.co.nz/archive/listener-nz-2011/the-rise-of-necrotising-fasciitis (accessed 16 March 2017).

13 Health Research Council of New Zealand, 'Coalition to Identify Potential Vaccines for Rheumatic Fever', 16 September 2014, www.hrc.govt.nz/news-and-media/media/coalition-identify-potential-vaccines-rheumatic-fever (accessed 16 March 2017).

14 D.A. Williamson et al., 'M-Protein Analysis of *Streptococcus pyogenes* Isolates Associated with Acute Rheumatic Fever in New Zealand', *J Clin Microbiol*, 53, 11 (2015), pp.3618–20, https://doi.org/10.1128/JCM.02129-15.

15 Irina Serdobova and Marie-Paule Kieny, 'Assembling a Global Vaccine Development Pipeline for Infectious Diseases in the Developing World', *Am J Public Health*, 96, 9 (2006), pp.1554–59, https://doi.org/10.2105/AJPH.2005.074583.

16 M.M. Struck, 'Vaccine R&D Success Rates and Development Times', *Nat Biotechnol*, 14, 5 (1996), pp.591–93.

17 D. A. Williamson et al., 'Increasing Incidence of Invasive Group A Streptococcus Disease in New Zealand, 2002–2012: A National Population-Based Study', *J Infect*, 70, 2 (2015), pp.127–34, https://doi.org/10.1016/j.jinf.2014.09.001.

18 D.K. Das, M.G. Baker and K. Venugopal, 'Increasing Incidence of Necrotizing Fasciitis in New Zealand: A Nationwide Study over the Period 1990 to 2006', *J Infect*, 63, 6 (2011), pp.429–33, https://doi.org/10.1016/j.jinf.2011.07.019.

19 Best Practice Advocacy Centre New Zealand, 'Rheumatic Fever in Māori: What Can

We Do Better?', *Best Practice Journal*, August 2011, www.bpac.org.nz/BPJ/2011/august/rheumatic.aspx (accessed 16 March 2017).

20. J.R. Oliver et al., 'Acute Rheumatic Fever and Exposure to Poor Housing Conditions in New Zealand: A Descriptive Study', *J Paediatr Child Health*, (2017), https://doi.org/10.1111/jpc.13421.

21. Hawke's Bay District Health Board, Our Health, 'Current Public Health Warnings and Alerts', www.ourhealthhb.nz/healthy-communities/current-public-health-warnings-and-alerts (accessed 16 March 2017).

22. Hawke's Bay District Health Board, 'Havelock North Campylobacter Outbreak Update – November 2016', www.ourhealthhb.nz/assets/News-and-Event-files/Gastro-update-flyer-Nov-A5.pdf (accessed 16 March 2017).

23. Institute of Environmental Science and Research (ESR), 'Interim Report on Genotype Analysis of Campylobacter Isolates', 19 August 2016, http://img.scoop.co.nz/media/pdfs/1608/Interim_Report_on_Campylobacter_genotyping__19Aug16.pdf (accessed 16 March 2017).

24. Department of Internal Affairs, 'Government Inquiry into Havelock North Drinking Water', www.dia.govt.nz/Government-Inquiry-into-Havelock-North-Drinking-Water (accessed 16 March 2017).

25. Public Health Surveillance, 'Annual Notifiable Disease Tables', https://surv.esr.cri.nz/surveillance/annual_diseasetables.php (accessed 16 March 2017).

26. D.A. Williamson et al., 'Genomic Insights into a Sustained National Outbreak of Yersinia pseudotuberculosis', *Genome Biol Evol*, 2017, https://doi.org/10.1093/gbe/evw285.

27. Public Health Surveillance, 'Sexually Transmitted Infections in New Zealand: Annual Surveillance Report 2014', https://surv.esr.cri.nz/surveillance/annual_sti.php?we_objectID=4248 (accessed 16 March 2017).

Chapter 3

1. Medical historians have found lots of references to the medical use of fungi stretching back thousands of years. Some of these seem to have involved eating mouldy foods

or applying them to wounds to cure infections. Backing up the written records, researchers have found traces of the antibiotic tetracycline in human bones from archaeological sites in Egypt and other countries.

2 A. Fleming, 'On the Antibacterial Action of Cultures of a Penicillium, with Special Reference to Their Use in the Isolation of *B. influenzae*', *Br J Exp Pathol*, 10, 3 (1929), pp.226–36, PMCID: PMC2048009.

3 D. J. Payne et al., 'Drugs for Bad Bugs: Confronting the Challenges of Antibacterial Discovery', *Nature Reviews Drug Discovery*, 6, 1 (2007), pp.29–40.

4 Review on Antimicrobial Resistance, 'Antibiotics in the Pipeline or Recently Licensed', https://amr-review.org/sites/default/files/Pipeline%20corrected-1_0.png (accessed 16 March 2017).

Chapter 4

1 WHO, *Antimicrobial Resistance: Global Report on Surveillance*, 2014.

2 Review on Antimicrobial Resistance, 'Tackling Drug-Resistant Infections Globally: Final Reports and Recommendations', 2016. This and other reports are available at: https://amr-review.org/Publications.html (accessed 16 March 2017).

3 Over the last few years, microbiologists have isolated antibiotic-resistant bacteria, or their genetic material, from layers of ancient soil and ice that have remained undisturbed for 5,000–30,000 years (see: G. G. Perron et al., 'Functional Characterization of Bacteria Isolated from Ancient Arctic Soil Exposes Diverse Resistance Mechanisms to Modern Antibiotics', *PLOS ONE*, 10, 3 (2015), e0069533; and V. M. D'Costa et al., 'Antibiotic Resistance is Ancient', *Nature*, 477, 7365 (2011), pp.457–61). Among the resistance genes discovered were ones that can also make bacteria resistant to amikacin, a modern semi-synthetic antibiotic that doesn't occur in nature. Just last year, researchers reported that a bacterium they isolated from a cave in New Mexico, US, was resistant to twenty-six of the forty antibiotics they tested (see: A. C. Pawlowski et al., 'A Diverse Intrinsic Antibiotic Resistome from a Cave

Bacterium', *Nat Commun*, 7 (2016), p.13803). The cave in question, Lechuguilla Cave, is an underground system more than 200 kilometres in size and 500 metres deep that has been isolated from the surface for over four million years. As well as having twelve resistance systems we know about, one bacterium they discovered, *Paenibacillus sp.* LC231, also had five ways of resisting antibiotics that we had never seen before.

Chapter 5

1. Center for Disease Dynamics, Economics & Policy, 'The State of the World's Antibiotics, 2015', CDDEP, Washington, D.C., 2015, https://cddep.org/sites/default/files/swa_2015_final.pdf (accessed 16 March 2017).

2. Review on Antimicrobial Resistance, 'Antimicrobials in Agriculture and the Environment: Reducing Unnecessary Use and Waste', December 2015, https://amr-review.org/sites/default/files/Antimicrobials%20in%20agriculture%20and%20the%20environment%20-%20Reducing%20unnecessary%20use%20and%20waste.pdf (accessed 16 March 2017).

3. T. P. Van Boeckela et al., 'Global Trends in Antimicrobial Use in Food Animals', *PNAS*, 112, 18 (2015), pp.5649–54.

4. A. H. Buschmann et al., 'Salmon Aquaculture and Antimicrobial Resistance in the Marine Environment', *PLOS ONE*, 7, 8 (2012), e42724.

5. P. E. Verweij et al., 'Azole Resistance in *Aspergillus fumigatus*: Can We Retain the Clinical Use of Moldactive Antifungal Azoles?', *Clin Infect Dis*, 62, 3 (2016), pp.362–68.

6. European Public Health Alliance & Changing Markets, 'Briefing: Drug Resistance Through the Back Door: How the Pharmaceutical Industry is Fuelling the Rise of Superbugs Through Pollution in Its Supply Chains', http://epha.org/wp-content/uploads/2016/08/DRUG-RESISTANCE-THROUGH-THE-BACK-DOOR_WEB.pdf (accessed 16 March 2017).

7. D. G. J. Larssona, C. de Pedroa and N. Paxeus, 'Effluent from Drug Manufactures Contains Extremely High Levels of Pharmaceuticals', *J Haz Mat*, 148, 3 (2007), pp.751–55.

8. International Federation

of Pharmaceutical Manufacturers & Associations, 'Industry Roadmap for Progress on Combating Antimicrobial Resistance – September 2016', www.ifpma.org/wp-content/uploads/2016/09/Roadmap-for-Progress-on-AMR-FINAL.pdf (accessed 16 March 2017).

Chapter 6

1. J.E. Hillerton et al., 'Use of Antimicrobials for Animals in New Zealand, and in Comparison with Other Countries', *NZ Vet J*, 65, 2 (2017), pp.71–77.

2. Ministry for Primary Industries, '2011–2014 Antibiotic Sales Analysis', MPI Technical Paper No: 2016/65, prepared for Systems Audit, Assurance & Monitoring Directorate by the Agricultural Compounds and Veterinary Medicines Group, October 2016, www.mpi.govt.nz/document-vault/14497 (accessed 16 March 2017).

3. A. Yoshii, H. Moriyama and T. Fukuhara, 'The Novel Kasugamycin 2'-N-acetyltransferase Gene aac(2')-IIa, Carried by the IncP Island, Confers Kasugamycin Resistance to Rice-Pathogenic Bacteria', *Appl Environ Microbiol*, 78, 16 (2012), pp.5555–64.

4. D.A. Williamson et al., 'Trends, Demographics and Disparities in Outpatient Antibiotic Consumption in New Zealand: A National Study', *J Antimicrob Chemother*, 71, 12 (2016), pp.3593–98.

5. P. Norris et al., 'Impact of Prescription Charges on People Living in Poverty: A Qualitative Study', *Res Social Adm Pharm*, 12, 6 (2016), pp.893–902.

6. P. Norris et al., 'Understanding and Use of Antibiotics amongst Samoan People in New Zealand', *J Prim Health Care*, 1, 1 (2009), pp.30–35.

7. Ministry of Health, 'The Health of New Zealand Adults 2011/12: Key Findings of the New Zealand Health Survey', December 2012, www.health.govt.nz/publication/health-new-zealand-adults-2011-12 (accessed 16 March 2017).

8. L. Ellison-Loschmann and N. Pearce, 'Improving Access to Health Care among New Zealand's Maori Population', *Am J Pub Health*, 96, 4 (2006), pp.612–17.

Chapter 7

1. D.A. Williamson and H. Heffernan, 'The Changing

Landscape of Antimicrobial Resistance in New Zealand', *NZ Med J*, 127, 1403 (2014), pp.41–54.

2 These strains produced a plasmid-encoded enzyme, called a penicillinase, that breaks penicillin's beta-lactam ring, essential for its antibiotic activity.

3 Like penicillin, methicillin inhibits the synthesis of bacterial cell walls by binding to bacterial enzymes known as penicillin-binding proteins (PBPs). The difference is that methicillin is not affected by penicillinase enzymes. These bacteria have picked up a gene called mecA that codes for a new PBP that binds very poorly to beta-lactam antibiotics. This means strains of *S. aureus* with a copy of mecA can still build their cell walls even when surrounded by beta-lactam antibiotics. The mecA gene is carried on a bit of genetic material that can move around, called the SCCmec. There are a number of different varieties of SCCmec but SCCmec-IV is becoming the most widespread. This might be because it doesn't seem to make *S. aureus* grow any slower, or be disadvantaged in any way.

4 D.A. Williamson et al., 'Clinical and Molecular Epidemiology of Methicillin-Resistant *Staphylococcus aureus* in New Zealand: Rapid Emergence of Sequence Type 5 (ST5)-SCCmec-IV as the Dominant Community-Associated MRSA Clone', *PLOS One*, 8, 4 (2013), e62020.

5 D.A. Williamson et al., 'High Usage of Topical Fusidic Acid and Rapid Clonal Expansion of Fusidic Acid-Resistant *Staphylococcus aureus*: A Cautionary Tale', *Clin Infect Dis*, 59, 10 (2014), pp.1451–54.

6 'US Woman Dies after Contracting Superbug That's Resistant to Every Available Antibiotic', *Stuff*, 13 January 2017, www.stuff.co.nz/world/americas/88410414/us-woman-dies-after-contracting-superbug-that's-resistant-to-every-available-antibiotic (accessed 16 March 2017).

7 L. Chen et al., 'Notes from the Field: Panresistant New Delhi Metallobeta- Lactamase-Producing *Klebsiella pneumoniae* – Washoe County, Nevada, 2016', *MMWR Morb Mortal Wkly Rep*, 66, 1 (2017), p.33, www.cdc.gov/mmwr/volumes/66/wr/mm6601a7.htm?s_cid=mm6601a7_w

8 Michelle Duff, 'Teacher NZ's First Victim of Superbug', Fairfax, 19 November 2013, www.stuff.co.nz/national/health/9414252/Teacher-NZs-first-victim-of-superbug (accessed 16 March 2017).

9 Kristin Dyet, Rosemary Woodhouse and Helen Heffernan, 'Annual Survey of Extended-Spectrum B-Lactamase (ESBL)-Producing Enterobacteriaceae, 2014', Antibiotic Reference Laboratory, ESR, July 2014, https://surv.esr.cri.nz/PDF_surveillance/Antimicrobial/ESBL/ESBL_2014.pdf (accessed 17 March 2017).

10 Public Health Surveillance, 'Acquired Carbapenemases in Enterobacteriaceae', https://surv.esr.cri.nz/antimicrobial/AccqEnterobacteriaceae.php (accessed 17 March 2017).

11 J. Creighton, H. Heffernan and J. Howard, 'Isolation of Seven Distinct Carbapenemase-Producing Gram-Negative Organisms from a Single Patient', *J Antimicrob Chemother*, 72, 1 (2017), pp.317–19.

12 G.C. Cerqueira et al., 'Multi-Institute Analysis of Carbapenem Resistance Reveals Remarkable Diversity, Unexplained Mechanisms, and Limited Clonal Outbreaks', *PNAS*, 114, 5 (2017), p.1135–40.

13 Y.Y. Liu et al., 'Emergence of Plasmid-mediated Colistin Resistance Mechanism MCR-1 in Animals and Human Beings in China: A Microbiological and Molecular Biological Study', *Lancet Infect Dis*, 16, 2 (2016), pp.161–68.

14 M.F. Kluytmans-van den Bergh, 'Presence of mcr-1-Positive *Enterobacteriaceae* in Retail Chicken Meat but not in Humans in the Netherlands since 2009', *Euro Surveill*, 21, 9 (2016), https://doi.org/10.2807/1560-7917.ES.2016.21.9.30149.

15 H. Fifer et al., 'Failure of Dual Antimicrobial Therapy in Treatment of Gonorrhea', *N Engl J Med*, 374, 25 (2016), pp.2504–6.

16 Helen Heffernan, Rosemary Woodhouse and Deborah Williamson, 'Antimicrobial Resistance and Molecular Epidemiology of *Neisseria gonorrhoeae* in New Zealand, 2014–15', FW15061, prepared for the Ministry of Health, ESR, December 2015, https://surv.esr.cri.nz/PDF_surveillance/

17 T.C. Clark et al., 'Youth'12 Overview: The Health and Wellbeing of New Zealand Secondary School Students in 2012', Youth2000 series, The University of Auckland, 2013, www.fmhs.auckland. ac.nz/assets/fmhs/faculty/ ahrg/docs/2012-overview.pdf (accessed 17 March 2017).

18 R.M.G.J. Houben and P.J. Dodd, 'The Global Burden of Latent Tuberculosis Infection: A Re-Estimation Using Mathematical Modelling', *PLOS Med*, 13, 10 (2016), e1002152.

19 University of Auckland, 'Auckland Contributes to TB Drug Development', 19 February 2015, www.auckland. ac.nz/en/about/news-events-and-notices/news/news-2015/02/auckland-contributes-to-tb-drug-development.html (accessed 17 March 2017).

20 T.L. Goh et al., 'Extensively Drug-Resistant Tuberculosis: New Zealand's First Case and the Challenges of Management in a Low-prevalence Country', *Med J Aust*, 194, 11 (2011), pp.602–4.

Chapter 8

1 Start by wetting your hands with clean running water. It doesn't matter if it's hot or cold. Then turn off the tap and lather your hands with soap. Make sure you lather the backs of your hands, your wrists, between your fingers and under your nails. There is no good evidence that normal healthy people need to use 'antibacterial' soaps. Not unless they are a healthcare professional at work. Scrub your hands for at least twenty seconds, then rinse well under clean running water. Now here's the really important bit: bacteria transfer more easily to and from wet hands so make sure you dry your hands thoroughly.

2 Child Poverty Monitor, 'Child Poverty Trends over Time, 2016', www.childpoverty. co.nz/sites/default/files/ ChildPovertyTrendsOver Time.pdf (accessed 17 March 2017).

3 UNICEF, 'Child Rights', www.unicef.org.nz/learn/our-focus-areas/child-rights (accessed 17 March 2017).

4 Expert Advisory Group on Solutions to Child Poverty, 'Solutions to Child Poverty in New Zealand: Evidence for

4. Action', December 2012, www.occ.org.nz/assets/Uploads/EAG/Final-report/Final-report-Solutions-to-child-poverty-evidence-for-action.pdf (accessed 17 March 2017).

5. Parliamentary Council Office, 'Residential Tenancies Amendment Bill, Government Bill 109-3', www.legislation.govt.nz/bill/government/2015/0109/latest/DLM6681409.html (accessed 17 March 2017).

6. Figure.NZ, 'New Zealand Resident Traveller Departures from Auckland Airport: By Selected Purpose of Travel', Statistics New Zealand, https://figure.nz/chart/0tBJ8ZrE5jhvSywA-AwhUecXYPZjJypxI (accessed 17 March 2017).

7. WHO, 'Global Action Plan on Antimicrobial Resistance', 2015, www.who.int/antimicrobial-resistance/publications/global-action-plan/en (accessed 17 March 2017).

8. Ministry of Health, 'Antimicrobial Resistance', www.health.govt.nz/our-work/diseases-and-conditions/antimicrobial-resistance (accessed 17 March 2017).

9. The SciFund Challenge, https://scifundchallenge.org (accessed 17 March 2017).

10. D. L. Herbert et al., 'On the Time Spent Preparing Grant Proposals: An Observational Study of Australian Researchers', *BMJ Open*, 3, 5 (2013), e002800.

11. J. Gush et al., 'The Effect of Public Funding on Research Output: the New Zealand Marsden Fund', NBER Working Paper No. 21652, October 2015, www.nber.org/papers/w21652 (accessed 17 March 2017).

12. Ministry of Business, Innovation and Employment, 'Science and Innovation System Performance Report', 2016, www.mbie.govt.nz/info-services/science-innovation/performance/document-image-library/2016-science-and-innovation-system-performance-report.pdf (accessed 17 March 2017).

13. Ministry of Business, Innovation and Employment, 'Endeavour Fund Investment Plan 2016–2019', August 2016, www.mbie.govt.nz/info-services/science-innovation/investment-funding/current-funding/2017-endeavour-round/

document-image-library/mbie-endeavour-fund-investment-plan-2016-2019.pdf (accessed 17 March 2017).

14. Professor Kurt Krause, personal communication.

15. Maurice Wilkins Centre for Molecular Biodiscovery, www.mauricewilkinscentre.org (accessed 17 March 2017).

16. Department of Health and Department for Environment, Food & Rural Affairs, 'UK Five Year Antimicrobial Resistance Strategy, 2013 to 2018', September 2013, www.gov.uk/government/uploads/system/uploads/attachment_data/file/244058/20130902_UK_5_year_AMR_strategy.pdf (accessed 17 March 2017).

17. Antibiotic Research UK, www.antibioticresearch.org.uk (accessed 17 March 2017).

18. Longitude Prize, https://longitudeprize.org (accessed 17 March 2017).

19. Office of the Minister of Science and Innovation, 'National Science Challenges', 2012, www.mbie.govt.nz/info-services/science-innovation/national-science-challenges/documents-image-library/key-documents/National-Science-Challenges-Cabinet-paper.pdf (accessed 17 March 2017).

20. 'The Great NZ Science Project', video, 11 November 2012, www.youtube.com/watch?v=SPampEgnYe8 (accessed 17 March 2017).

21. Steven Joyce, 'Public to Have Say on NZ Science Challenges', Beehive.govt.nz, 8 November 2012, www.beehive.govt.nz/release/public-have-say-nz-science-challenges (accessed 17 March 2017).

22. 'Fighting Disease', video, 10 November 2012, www.youtube.com/watch?v=8J_B2c5kUMw (accessed 17 March 2017).

23. Steven Joyce, 'National Science Challenge Panel Appointed', Beehive.govt.nz, 7 February 2013, www.beehive.govt.nz/release/national-science-challenge-panel-appointed (accessed 17 March 2017).

24. Peak Panel, 'Report of National Science Challenges Panel', March 2013, www.pmcsa.org.nz/wp-content/uploads/Report-of-National-Science-Challenges.pdf (accessed 17 March 2017).

25. Steven Joyce, 'Budget 2013: National Science Challenges Announced – Budget Boost of $73.5m', Beehive.govt.nz,

1 May 2013, www.beehive.govt.nz/release/budget-2013-national-science-challenges-announced-budget-boost-735m (accessed 17 March 2017).

26 Ministry of Business, Innovation and Employment, 'National Science Challenges: Potential Challenges for Consideration by Peak Panel: Health, Demographic Change and Wellbeing', February 2013, www.mbie.govt.nz/info-services/science-innovation/national-science-challenges/documents-image-library/key-documents/Potential-challenges-peak-panel-Health-demographic-change-wellbeing.pdf (accessed 17 March 2017).

27 As a side project, I've curated a number of pop-up science-art exhibitions in which I challenge artists/illustrators to each make a work of art using a solution of harmless glowing bacteria and a collection of large Petri dishes. Wherever the artists 'paint' with the bacteria they will grow, and wherever they grow they will glow. We've taken photographs of all the works from the various exhibitions and put the images onto a range of merchandise, including T-shirts, notebooks, mugs and bags. All profits go to my lab to help pay for our research. See: www.redbubble.com/people/siouxsiew.

28 Auckland University have set up a website so that people can contribute to our search for new antibiotics. It costs us about $250 to test each fungus, and we've over nine thousand fungi to test, so every donation, no matter how small, makes a difference. We send all donors updates of our progress. Donors that contribute $250 or more are also sent a certificate and picture of the fungus they have 'adopted'. See: www.giving.auckland.ac.nz/fungi.

ABOUT THE AUTHOR

Dr Siouxsie Wiles is an award-winning scientist and communicator who has made a career of manipulating nasty microbes. In a nutshell, Siouxsie and her team make nasty bacteria glow in the dark to better understand how they cause disease and to find new medicines. Siouxsie studied medical microbiology at the University of Edinburgh, UK and then did a PhD in microbiology at the Centre for Ecology and Hydrology in Oxford. She spent several years working at Imperial College London where her research culminated in winning the inaugural UK National Centre for the Replacement, Refinement and Reduction of Animals in Research prize. In 2009, Siouxsie was awarded a Sir Charles Hercus Fellowship from the Health Research Council of New Zealand and relocated to the University of Auckland. Siouxsie has a keen interest in demystifying science for the public and has won numerous prizes for her efforts, including the Prime Minister's Science Media Communication Prize and the Royal Society of New Zealand Callaghan Medal. In 2016, Siouxsie was named a Blake Leader by the Sir Peter Blake Leadership Trust.

ACKNOWLEDGEMENTS

I'd like to dedicate this book to a very special little girl whose struggle with MRSA has turned my intellectual curiosity for infectious microbes into a passionate quest to find new antibiotics.

I would not have been able to write this book without the patience and support of my husband Steven, daughter Eve, and my mum and dad, Graham and Hazel, who tolerated my spending the summer holiday locked away in the office. Thank you. Thanks also to my wider whānau for all their support and encouragement.

Massive thanks to Sam Moller, Heather Hendrickson, Jo Richdale and Geoff Walker and the rest of the BWB Texts team, for whipping my manuscript into a readable book. Thank you also to readers Kurt Krause and Shaun Hendy for your helpful and thoughtful comments.

I would like to thank all the members, past and present, of the Bioluminescent Superbugs Lab for their hard work, dedication and passion. Special mention must go to Benedict Uy, Hannah Read and Jimmy Dalton for putting up with all my crazy ideas over the last few years.

Finally, I would also like to thank the people who have turned me into the scientist I am today and those who continue to support me: Marc

Bailey, Laura Bennet, Michelle Dickinson, Richard Easther, Gad Frankel, Nicola Gaston, Michelle Glass, John Fraser, Kate Hannah, Shaun Hendy, John Hosking, Phil Hill, Andy Lilley, Cate Macinnis-Ng, Brian Robertson, Shiranee Sriskandan, Simon Swift, Andy Whiteley and Douglas Young.

About BWB Texts

BWB Texts are short books on big subjects: succinct narratives spanning history, memoir, contemporary issues, science and more from great New Zealand writers. All BWB Texts are available digitally, with selected works also in paperback. New Texts are published monthly – please visit www.bwb.co.nz to see the latest releases.

BWB Texts include:

Hopes Dashed?: The Economics of Gender Inequality
Prue Hyman

Safeguarding the Future: Governing in an Uncertain World
Jonathan Boston

The Stolen Island: Searching for 'Ata
Scott Hamilton

The Post-Snowden Era: Mass Surveillance and Privacy in New Zealand
Kathleen Kuehn

The Bike and Beyond: Life on Two Wheels in Aotearoa New Zealand
Laura Williamson

Late Love: Sometimes Doctors Need Saving as Much as Their Patients
Glenn Colquhoun

Three Cities: Seeking Hope in the Anthropocene
Rod Oram

Playing for Both Sides: Love Across the Tasman
Stephanie Johnson

Complacent Nation
Gavin Ellis

The First Migration: Māori Origins 3000BC – AD1450
Atholl Anderson

Silencing Science
Shaun Hendy

Going Places: Migration, Economics and the Future of New Zealand
Julie Fry & Hayden Glass

The Interregnum: Rethinking New Zealand
Morgan Godfery (ed)

Christchurch Ruptures
Katie Pickles

Home Truths: Confronting New Zealand's Housing Crisis
Philippa Howden-Chapman

Polluted Inheritance: New Zealand's Freshwater Crisis
Mike Joy

Wealth and New Zealand
Max Rashbrooke

Why Science Is Sexist
Nicola Gaston

Towards a Warmer World: What Climate Change Will Mean for New Zealand's Future
Veronika Meduna

The Edge of Life: Controversies and Challenges in Human Health
Mike Berridge

Out of the Vaipe, the Deadwater: A Writer's Early Life
Albert Wendt

No Country for Old Maids?: Talking About the 'Man Drought'
Hannah August

Time of Useful Consciousness: Acting Urgently on Climate Change
Ralph Chapman

Generation Rent: Rethinking New Zealand's Priorities
Shamubeel & Selena Eaqub

Haerenga: Early Māori Journeys Across the Globe
Vincent O'Malley

On Coming Home
Paula Morris

Ruth, Roger and Me: Debts and Legacies
Andrew Dean

The Struggle for Sovereignty: New Zealand and Twenty-First Century Statehood
Margaret Wilson

The Child Poverty Debate: Myths, Misconceptions and Misunderstandings
Jonathan Boston & Simon Chapple

The Piketty Phenomenon: New Zealand Perspectives
Various

Barefoot Years
Martin Edmond

New Myths and Old Politics: The Waitangi Tribunal and the Challenge of Tradition
Tipene O'Regan